TRAVELER'S HEALTH AND SAFETY

SOURCEBOOK

SECOND EDITION

Health Reference Series

TRAVELER'S HEALTH AND SAFETY
SOURCEBOOK
SECOND EDITION

Basic Consumer Health and Safety Information for Travelers, Including Types of Travel, Tips on Choosing the Right Travel Accommodations, Pretravel Preparations, and Common Travel-Related Illnesses

Along with Safety Measures during Travel and at the Destination, a Glossary of Terms Related to Travel Health, and a Directory of Resources for Additional Help and Information

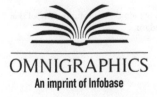

OMNIGRAPHICS
An imprint of Infobase

Bibliographic Note

Because this page cannot legibly accommodate all the copyright notices,
the Bibliographic Note portion of the Preface constitutes an extension
of the copyright notice.

* * *

OMNIGRAPHICS
An imprint of Infobase
8 The Green
Suite #19225
Dover, DE 19901
www.infobase.com
James Chambers, *Editorial Director*

* * *

Copyright © 2024 Infobase
ISBN 978-0-7808-2146-0
E-ISBN 978-0-7808-2147-7

Library of Congress Cataloging-in-Publication Data

Names: Chambers, James (Editor), editor.

Title: Traveler's health and safety sourcebook / edited by James Chambers.

Description: Second edition. | Dover, DE: Omnigraphics, an imprint of Infobase, [2024] | Series: Health reference series | Includes index. | Summary: "Provides basic health and safety information for travelers, covering various types of travel, modes of transportation, accommodation options, common travel illnesses, preparation tips, and safety measures during travel and at destinations. Includes an index, glossary of related terms, and other resources"-- Provided by publisher.

Identifiers: LCCN 2024017330 (print) | LCCN 2024017331 (ebook) | ISBN 9780780821460 (library binding) | ISBN 9780780821477 (ebook)

Subjects: LCSH: Travel--Health aspects.

Classification: LCC RA783.5 .T678 2024 (print) | LCC RA783.5 (ebook) | DDC 613.6/8--dc23/eng/20240607

LC record available at https://lccn.loc.gov/2024017330

LC ebook record available at https://lccn.loc.gov/2024017331

Table of Contents

Part 8. Additional Help and Information

Preface

ABOUT THIS BOOK

Traveling offers a wonderful opportunity to meet new people, explore different cultures, and broaden one's perspective on the world. Whether for education, business, tourism, or pilgrimage, traveling provides many exciting experiences and can serve as an excellent stress reliever. However, traveling also presents various health and safety risks, making it crucial to take proper precautions.

Traveler's Health and Safety Sourcebook, Second Edition provides comprehensive information on travel health, safety advisories, and different types of travel. It covers health risks associated with travel, including bacterial, viral, fungal, and parasitic infections, as well as conditions such as jet lag, food poisoning, motion sickness, and altitude illness. The book offers guidelines on staying safe and maintaining health during travel, at your destination, and after returning home. It concludes with a glossary of terms related to travel health and a directory of resources for further help and support.

HOW TO USE THIS BOOK

This book is divided into parts and chapters. Parts focus on broad areas of interest. Chapters are devoted to single topics within a part.

Part 1: Introduction to Travel Health and Safety offers an overview of travel and tourism, focusing on essential travel safety and security tips, travel advisories, and a traveler's checklist. It also addresses frequently asked questions related to traveler health and safety during and after travel.

Part 2: Types of Travel explores various forms of travel, including traveling abroad for the holidays, studying abroad, business, faith-based, and long-term travel. It also covers specialized types of travel, such as adventure travel and travel to high-risk areas.

Part 3: Health Risks during Travel provides detailed information on diseases and infections that travelers may encounter, including bacterial, viral, fungal, and parasitic infections. Other health risks such as altitude illness, blood clots, jet lag, and sun exposure are discussed. Preventive measures and tips for managing these risks are also discussed.

Part 4: Modes of Travel and Shelters discusses different modes of travel, including cruise safety, chartered flights, and road safety. It also provides guidance on choosing safe tourist accommodations and offers information on hosting a foreign exchange student and hotel safety.

Part 5: Pretravel Preparations covers crucial aspects of travel preparation, including obtaining travel insurance, necessary vaccinations, and assembling a travel health kit. It offers practical advice for ensuring a safe and healthy trip.

Part 6: Travelers with Special Needs focuses on health and safety considerations for travelers with specific needs, including pregnant women, older adults, immunocompromised individuals, and others. It offers tailored advice for these groups to ensure a safe travel experience.

Part 7: Safety and Security Measures discusses customs and import regulations, cybersecurity tips for international travelers, procedures for handling lost or stolen passports abroad, and dealing with legal issues such as arrest or detention during travel. It also covers safety measures in the event of a death during travel.

Part 8: Additional Help and Information includes a glossary of terms related to travel health and safety and a directory of resources for further support and information.

BIBLIOGRAPHIC NOTE

This volume contains documents and excerpts from publications issued by the following U.S. government agencies: Bureau of Consular Affairs; Centers for Disease Control and Prevention (CDC); Federal Communications Commission (FCC); Federal Trade Commission (FTC); International Trade Administration (ITA); National Park Service (NPS); Ready.gov; Transportation Security Administration (TSA); U.S. Bureau of Labor Statistics (BLS); U.S. Department of Commerce (DOC); U.S. Department of Education (ED); U.S. Department of Health and Human Services (HHS); U.S. Department of State (DOS); U.S. Department of Transportation (DOT); and USA.gov.

ABOUT THE *HEALTH REFERENCE SERIES*

The *Health Reference Series* is designed to provide basic medical information for patients, families, caregivers, and the general public. Each volume provides comprehensive coverage on a particular topic. This is especially important for people who may be dealing with a newly diagnosed disease or a chronic disorder in themselves or in a family member. People looking for preventive guidance, information about disease warning signs, medical statistics, and risk factors for health problems will also find answers to their questions in the *Health Reference Series*. The *Series*, however, is not intended to serve as a tool for diagnosing illness, in prescribing treatments, or as a substitute for the physician-patient relationship. All people concerned about medical symptoms or the possibility of disease are encouraged to seek professional care from an appropriate health-care provider.

A NOTE ABOUT SPELLING AND STYLE

Health Reference Series editors use *Stedman's Medical Dictionary* as an authority for questions related to the spelling of medical terms and *The Chicago Manual of Style* for questions related to grammatical structures, punctuation, and other editorial concerns. Consistent adherence is not always possible, however, because the individual volumes within the *Series* include many documents from a wide variety of different producers, and the editor's primary goal is to present material from each source as accurately as is possible. This sometimes means that information in different chapters or sections may follow other guidelines and alternate spelling authorities. For example, occasionally a copyright holder may require that eponymous terms be shown in possessive forms (Crohn's disease vs. Crohn disease) or that British spelling norms be retained (leukaemia vs. leukemia).

HEALTH REFERENCE SERIES UPDATE POLICY

The inaugural book in the *Health Reference Series* was the first edition of *Cancer Sourcebook* published in 1989. Since then, the *Series* has been enthusiastically received by librarians and in the medical community. In order to maintain the standard of providing high-quality health information for the layperson, the editorial staff felt it was necessary to implement a policy of updating volumes when warranted.

Medical researchers have been making tremendous strides, and it is the purpose of the *Health Reference Series* to stay current with the most recent advances. Each decision to update a volume is made on an individual basis. Some of the considerations include how much new information is available and the feedback we receive from people who use the books. If there is a topic you would like to see added to the update list, or an area of medical concern you feel has not been adequately addressed, please write to: custserv@infobaselearning.com.

Part 1 | Introduction to Travel Health and Safety

Chapter 1 | Key Sectors and Health Concerns in U.S. Travel and Tourism

According to the National Travel and Tourism Office (NTTO), the U.S. travel and tourism industry generated almost $1.9 trillion in economic output in 2019, supporting 9.2 million U.S. jobs. Travel and tourism exports accounted for 9 percent of all U.S. exports and 27 percent of all U.S. services exports. That same year, U.S. travel and tourism output represented 2.9 percent of gross domestic product (GDP). Expenditures by international visitors in the United States were $233.5 billion in 2019, with almost two-thirds of spending going toward personal expenditures, such as health ($1.2 billion) and education ($44.0 billion).

INDUSTRY SUBSECTORS AND EMPLOYMENT TRENDS IN TRAVEL AND TOURISM

Accommodations

In 2019, almost $14.1 billion of foreign direct investment (FDI) was invested in the accommodations industry worldwide. The year before, foreign-owned businesses employed 44,000 workers in the accommodations industry out of a total of 2.05 million employees in December 2018. According to U.S. employment figures, there were 1.4 million employees in the accommodations industry in December 2020. There were also 68,375 establishments in the accommodations industry across the United States in 2017.

The most common occupations in the industry are maids and housekeeping cleaners and hotel, motel, and resort desk clerks. In

2019, 473,010 maids and housekeeping cleaners were employed in the accommodations industry, earning an average annual wage of $26,540. For hotel, motel, and resort desk clerks, 251,050 people were employed in the industry, earning an average annual wage of $25,850.

Food Services and Drinking Places

In 2019, almost $44.7 billion was invested from around the world in the U.S. food services and drinking places industry, and foreign-owned businesses employed 614,400 people out of a total of 12.0 million employees in this industry in 2018. According to employment figures, 9.0 million people were employed in the food services and drinking places industry in December 2020. In 2017, there were 657,792 establishments in the hospitality industry, which includes food services and drinking places.

The most common occupations in the food services and drinking places industry are cooks and food preparation workers, as well as food and beverage serving workers. In 2019, there were over 2.4 million cooks and food preparation workers, with over 1.9 million cooks and almost 500,000 food preparation workers. Cooks earned an average annual wage of $26,990, and food preparation workers earned an average annual wage of $24,930. For food and beverage serving workers, there were over 6.1 million people employed in 2019, of which 2.2 million were waiters and waitresses. All food and beverage serving workers in the industry earned an average annual wage of $24,610, and waiters and waitresses earned an average annual wage of $26,530.

Air Transportation

There was $158 million in foreign direct investment into the U.S. air transportation industry in 2019, and foreign-owned businesses in the air transportation industry employed between 5,000 and 9,999 workers in 2018 out of a total employment of 497,800 in the industry. According to employment figures, there were 391,700 employees in the air transportation industry in December 2020. As of 2017, there were 4,441 establishments in the air transportation industry.

The most common occupations in the air transportation industry are airline pilots, copilots, and flight engineers; reservation and transportation ticket agents and travel clerks; and aircraft mechanics and service technicians. In 2019, 74,310 people were employed as airline pilots, copilots, and flight engineers in the air transportation industry, earning an average annual wage of $178,120. There were also 63,670 people employed as reservation and transportation ticket agents and travel clerks, earning an average annual wage of $50,140. Finally, there were 38,690 aircraft mechanics and service technicians in the air transportation industry in 2019, earning an average annual wage of $81,630.[1]

HEALTH AND DISEASE PATTERNS IN TRAVELERS
The Role of Travelers in Disease Spread

Travelers are an important population because of their mobility, their potential for exposure to infectious diseases outside their home country, and the possibility that they could bring those diseases from one country to another. The coronavirus 2019 (COVID-19) pandemic is the most recent example of the role travelers can play in the global spread of infectious diseases. Ebola virus, Zika virus, and antimicrobial-resistant pathogens are other examples of health threats whose geographic distribution has been facilitated by international travelers over the past several years. Travelers should be included in general and targeted epidemiologic surveillance—including the use of molecular genomic approaches—to better understand both the exposure risk and the effort of current and novel prevention recommendations.

Importance of Epidemiologic Surveillance

The ability to provide appropriate pretravel guidance—and, when necessary, optimal posttravel evaluation and treatment—is predicated on understanding the epidemiologic features (disease patterns) among different traveling populations. Accounting for behaviors that can influence and potentially increase risk for travel-associated infections and diseases (e.g., attendance at a mass gathering, long-term or adventure travel, visiting friends and family) helps the astute

---

[1] International Trade Administration (ITA), "Industry Overview," U.S. Department of Commerce (DOC), August 5, 2022. Available online. URL: www.trade.gov/selectusa-travel-tourism-hospitality-industry. Accessed July 26, 2024.

clinician make directed travel health recommendations and focus their attention on the more likely diagnoses from among the lengthy list of travel-associated infections and diseases. An understanding of the epidemiology of the diseases themselves, including modes of transmission, incubation periods, signs and symptoms, duration of infectiousness, and accuracy of diagnostic testing, is also crucial. Including international travelers in epidemiologic surveillance provides additional information about the presence, frequency, seasonality, and geographic distribution of diseases, which might shift over time due to outbreaks, changes in climate and vector habitat, emergence or reemergence in new areas or populations, successful public health interventions, or other factors.

Challenges in Assessing Travel-Related Infection Risk

The risk for travel-related infection can, however, be difficult to ascertain precisely for several reasons. Existing information regarding disease risk for travelers is limited because of the difficulty in obtaining accurate numerators (i.e., number of cases of infection among travelers) and denominators (i.e., number of overall travelers or number of travelers to a specific destination who are susceptible to infection). In cases of mild illness, travelers might never seek health care, or clinicians might not perform diagnostic tests to identify the cause. Travelers often visit multiple destinations, complicating identification of the location of exposure. Data on disease incidence in local populations might be available, but the relevance of such data to travelers—who have different risk behaviors, eating habits, accommodations, knowledge of and access to preventive measures, and activities—might be limited. In addition, epidemiologic investigations involving travelers use various methodologic designs, each with their own strengths and weaknesses, making findings difficult to compare or combine. Many single-clinic or single-destination investigations draw conclusions that might not be generalizable to travelers from different local, national, or cultural backgrounds.

Existing Epidemiologic Networks

Two existing networks provide epidemiologic data on international travelers from the United States and acquisition of travel-related illness. The GeoSentinel Global Surveillance Network is a worldwide data collection and communication network composed of International Society of Travel Medicine (ISTM)–associated travel and tropical medicine clinics that collect posttravel illness surveillance data. GeoSentinel scientists analyze these data to describe travel-related illness in specific populations of travelers.

Global TravEpiNet (GTEN) is a consortium of health clinics across the United States that deliver pretravel health consultations. Data from GTEN provide a snapshot of travelers seeking pretravel health care and longitudinal cohort data on risk for and acquisition of travel-associated conditions, including for a subset of travelers who self-collect biological samples for microbiologic and genomic testing.

Advancements in Travel Medicine Research

These travel medicine networks, and travel medicine researchers, increasingly are implementing next-generation sequencing tools to delineate the epidemiology of travel-associated infections and the role of travelers in the global spread of infectious diseases. Advances in the field of genomic sequencing enable high-resolution surveillance that can identify previously unrecognized geographic and epidemiologic associations. These molecular tools are becoming essential to understanding the spread of disease, the emergence of new pathogens or variants of existing ones, and the evolution of antimicrobial resistance. Combining these molecular techniques with traditional surveillance, epidemiologic approaches, and community-based participatory research represents a promising approach to expanding the evidence base underpinning the guidance and recommendations in the field of travel medicine. A broader evidence base will enable better-informed pretravel preparation for the individual traveler and the development of new approaches to mitigating the effort of travel on the global spread of disease.[2]

---

[2] "Disease Patterns in Travelers," Centers for Disease Control and Prevention (CDC), May 1, 2023. Available online. URL: wwwnc.cdc.gov/travel/yellowbook/2024/introduction/disease-patterns-in-travelers. Accessed July 26, 2024.

TRAVEL AND TOURISM

The NTTO creates a positive climate for growth in travel and tourism by reducing institutional barriers to tourism, administering joint marketing efforts, providing official travel and tourism statistics, and coordinating efforts across federal agencies through the Tourism Policy Council (TPC). The office works to enhance the international competitiveness of the U.S. travel and tourism industry and increase its exports, thereby creating U.S. employment and economic growth through:

- management of the travel and tourism statistical system for assessing the economic contribution of the industry and providing the sole source for characteristic statistics on international travel to and from the United States
- design and administration of export expansion activities
- development and management of tourism policy, strategy, and advocacy
- technical assistance for expanding this key export (international tourism) and assisting in domestic economic development[3]

WHAT THE INTERNATIONAL TRADE ADMINISTRATION DOES FOR YOU

- promote U.S. policies that encourage the competitiveness of the U.S. travel industry
- provide business counseling, match-making, and promotional support services to help U.S. destinations and attractions penetrate new markets and increase market share
- seek to ensure that U.S. regulations and other programs do not adversely affect U.S. industry competitiveness
- provide information, trade data, and market analysis to the U.S. travel industry, partners, and policymakers

---

[3] "Travel and Tourism," U.S. Department of Commerce (DOC), August 29, 2023. Available online. URL: www.commerce.gov/tags/travel-and-tourism. Accessed July 26, 2024.

- maintain close relationships with the U.S. travel industry to focus and construct programs that enhance the industry's competitiveness and overseas profile[4]

---

[4] International Trade Administration (ITA), "Travel and Tourism Industry," U.S. Department of Commerce (DOC), January 25, 2020. Available online. URL: www.trade.gov/travel-tourism-industry. Accessed July 26, 2024.

Chapter 2 | Travel Safety and Security

Chapter Contents

STAYING SAFE AND HEALTHY DURING TRAVEL

Take steps during travel to stay safe and healthy and avoid experiences that might ruin your trip.

Wash Your Hands

Regular handwashing is one of the best ways to remove germs, avoid getting sick, and prevent the spread of germs to others. Wash your hands and take other precautions to prevent getting and spreading diseases while traveling:

- Wash your hands with soap and water. If soap and water are not available, use hand sanitizer containing at least 60 percent alcohol.
- Avoid touching your eyes, nose, or mouth with unwashed hands. If you need to touch your face, make sure your hands are clean.
- Cover your mouth and nose with a tissue or your sleeve (not your hands) when you cough or sneeze.
- Avoid contact with people who are sick.
- If you get sick during travel, stay in your accommodations, unless you need medical care.

Choose Safe Transportation

Motor vehicle crashes are a leading cause of death among travelers. In many middle- or low-income destinations, there may be poor road surfaces, roads without shoulders, unprotected curves and cliffs, or no streetlights. In some destinations, traffic laws and road signs may not be regularly followed. Follow these tips to reduce your risk of getting injured:

- Always wear a seat belt.
- Do not drive at night, especially in unfamiliar or rural areas.
- Do not ride motorcycles. If you must ride a motorcycle, wear a helmet.
- Know local traffic laws before you get behind the wheel.

- Do not drink and drive.
- Only ride in marked taxis that have seat belts.
- Avoid overcrowded, overweight, or top-heavy buses or vans.
- Be alert when crossing the street, especially in countries where people drive on the left.

Prevent Bug Bites

On your trip, use insect repellent and take other steps to avoid bug bites. Bugs, including mosquitoes, ticks, fleas, and flies, can spread diseases, such as malaria, yellow fever, Zika, dengue, chikungunya, and Lyme disease.

- Use an Environmental Protection Agency (EPA)-registered insect repellent with one of the following active ingredients: DEET, picaridin, IR3535, oil of lemon eucalyptus (OLE), para-menthane-diol (PMD), or 2-undecanone.
- Always apply sunscreen first, let it dry, and then apply insect repellent. Follow the label instructions and reapply both as directed.
- Wear long-sleeved shirts and long pants when outdoors.

Choose Safe Food and Drinks

Contaminated food or drinks can cause travelers' diarrhea and other diseases, disrupting your travel. Travelers to low- or middle-income destinations are especially at risk. Choose safer food and drinks to prevent getting sick.

- Eat foods that have been fully cooked and served hot.
- Do not eat fresh vegetables or fruits unless you can wash or peel them yourself.
- Drink only bottled, sealed beverages, and avoid ice—it was likely made with tap water.

Avoid Animals

Animals can look cute and cuddly, but they can spread disease and may be dangerous. When traveling, do not pet or feed animals, even pets, as they may not be vaccinated against rabies and other diseases. Animal bites can cause bacterial infections that may require antibiotics, so seek medical attention after any animal encounter. Also, be sure you are up-to-date on your tetanus vaccination.

Protect against Sun and Extreme Temperatures

Apply sunscreen with sun protection factor 15 (SPF 15) or higher when traveling. Protecting yourself from the sun is not just for tropical beaches—you can get a sunburn even if it is cloudy or cold.

- If you are traveling in hot weather or in a hot climate, wear loose, lightweight, light-colored clothing.
- When traveling in cold weather or climates, wear warm clothing in several loose layers.

Emergencies and Natural Disasters

If you or a travel companion gets an injury or sickness that cannot be helped with basic first aid or an over-the-counter (OTC) medicine, seek medical attention right away. Visit Getting Health Care During Travel (wwwnc.cdc.gov/travel/page/health-care-during-travel) to learn how to connect with a doctor or medical services during your trip.

If you bought evacuation insurance and think you need to use it, call the travel insurance company for assistance.

For other emergencies or natural disasters, you may want to do the following:

- Contact family, friends, a trusted colleague, or your employer as soon as possible after the disaster to inform them of your location and health status.
- Monitor Travel Advisories and announcements by the U.S. Department of State (DOS; https://travel.state.gov/content/travel/en/international-travel.html) and the Voice of America (VOA) websites.
- Contact the U.S. Embassy or Consulate.[1]

---

[1] "During Travel," Centers for Disease Control and Prevention (CDC), June 15, 2021. Available online. URL: wwwnc.cdc.gov/travel/page/health-during-trip. Accessed July 26, 2024.

AFTER TRAVEL TIPS

You may get infected during travel but not have symptoms until you get home. If you recently traveled and feel sick, particularly with a fever, talk to your health-care provider and tell them about your travel.

Contact Your Health-Care Provider If You Feel Sick

Contact your health-care provider if you feel sick after your trip. Sharing the following information may help your health-care provider identify possible diseases or infections:

- your vaccination history
- where you traveled
- your reasons for traveling
- your travel activities, including swimming, hiking, and so on
- the timeframe of your vacation
- where you stayed, such as hotels, family or friends' homes, hostels, or tents
- what you ate and drank
- animals you had close contact with or touched
- if you have any injuries, scratches, or bug bites
- health care or medications you received during your trip
- close contact with other people, including sexual encounters
- if you got any tattoos or piercings

If your health-care provider has trouble determining why you are feeling sick, you may want to ask to speak with an infectious disease doctor or travel medicine specialist. Find a clinic for a travel medicine specialist.

Long-Term Travelers

Long-term travelers, such as expatriate workers, Peace Corps volunteers, or missionaries, have a greater risk of getting infected, sometimes without symptoms, during travel. If you are a long-term traveler, consider having a thorough medical exam or interview

16

with your health-care provider after you return to the United States.[2]

Section 2.2 | Crisis Preparedness and Safety for Travelers

Whether traveling or living outside the United States, there are ways to prepare for a potential crisis.

BE INFORMED

Thoroughly review the Traveler's Checklist (https://travel.state. gov/content/travel/en/international-travel/before-you-go/ travelers-checklist.html) page, which provides details on the Smart Traveler Enrollment Plan, Travel Advisories, emergency assistance, medical care, insurance, and more.

BE PREPARED

- Have plenty of food and drinking water available in case of a crisis.
- Ensure you have supplies for young children, such as diapers, formula, and baby food.
- Have at least five days' worth of medication on hand and keep your prescription handy.
- If you rely on assistive medical devices, have a backup power supply for your device in case of a power outage.
- Your emergency kit should also include your passports, birth certificates for overseas children, cash in the local currency, a card with local translations of basic terms, and an electrical current converter.
- If you have pets, ensure you have their food, supplies, and vaccination records.

---

[2] "After Travel Tips," Centers for Disease Control and Prevention (CDC), May 22, 2021. Available online. URL: wwwnc.cdc.gov/travel/page/after-trip. Accessed July 26, 2024.

BE CONNECTED

- Keep a list of your emergency contacts handy and create a communication plan for reaching family and friends during a crisis.
- Consider alternative ways to communicate if phone lines are affected during a crisis. Update your social media status often and send messages regularly to let friends and family know how you are doing.
- Many U.S. Embassies and Consulates, along with the Bureau of Consular Affairs (BCA), use social media to provide information—connect with them through Twitter and Facebook.

BE SAFE

- Have an exit strategy and know more than one way to get to safety without relying on assistance. A crisis event may make some roads impassable or unsafe and may prevent or delay emergency responders.
- Follow instructions from local authorities and monitor local radio, television, social media, and other sources for updates.
- If you are staying in a hotel, familiarize yourself with the hotel's emergency plan for various crisis events, such as fire, flood, electrical outage, storms, and so on.
- Keep in touch with hotel staff as well as your tour operators, airline, or cruise company, and local officials for instructions.
- Contact the nearest U.S. Embassies and Consulates if you need emergency help. Note that this will not alert emergency responders. If you need emergency medical attention or police assistance, contact local authorities directly if possible.
- Learn about your destination and potential risks of traveling there on the Country Information Pages (https://travel.state.gov/content/travel/en/international-travel/International-Travel-Country-Information-Pages.html), Ready.gov (www.ready.gov),

and the Centers for Disease Control and Prevention (CDC; www.cdc.gov) websites.[1]

TRAVEL AND NATURAL DISASTERS

Consider these tips to prepare and protect yourself in the event of a natural disaster:

- Natural disasters, such as hurricanes, floods, tsunamis, tornadoes, or earthquakes, can occur while you are on a trip. They can seriously injure large numbers of people, spread diseases, disrupt sanitation, and interrupt normal public services.
- Be familiar with the risks of natural disasters at your destination and local warning systems, evacuation routes, and shelters.

If a Natural Disaster Strikes

- Follow instructions provided by local emergency and public health authorities. U.S. travelers visiting other countries can also seek advice from the nearest U.S. Embassy.
- Be aware of your surroundings and avoid hazards:
  - Stay away from wild or stray animals.
  - Do not use electric tools or appliances while standing in water.
  - Avoid swiftly moving water during floods.
  - Prevent carbon monoxide poisoning by only using generators or other gasoline-, propane-, natural gas-, or charcoal-burning devices outside and away from open windows, doors, and air vents.

During the Aftermath

- Be aware of the risks for injury during and after a natural disaster. After a natural disaster, deaths are most often due to blunt trauma, crush-related injuries, or drowning.

---

[1] Bureau of Consular Affairs, "Crisis and Disaster Abroad: Be Ready," U.S. Department of State (DOS), February 22, 2024. Available online. URL: https://travel.state.gov/content/travel/en/international-travel/before-you-go/crisis_and_disaster_abroad_be_ready.html. Accessed July 26, 2024.

- Be careful during clean-up. Avoid downed power lines, electrical outlets exposed to water, and interrupted gas lines.
- Eat and drink only safe food and water.
- Seek medical care if you are injured, sick, or having trouble coping with stress.

The best way for travelers to stay healthy and safe when journeying to a new place is to plan ahead and stay well-informed. Know your destination's risk for natural disasters before you book your trip.[2]

Section 2.3 | Safety and Security for U.S. Citizens Traveling Abroad

RISKS AND SAFETY MEASURES

U.S. citizens traveling abroad face a wide range of risks not generally prevalent in the United States. These risks include sanitation issues (e.g., nonpotable water), increased risk for traffic accidents due to poor road conditions and unfamiliarity with local norms, local insect-borne illness or disease vectors, injury from adventure tourism or overexposure to unfamiliar climates, and violence ranging from petty theft to terrorism.

Challenges in Seeking Help Abroad

Travelers going overseas, particularly tourists, can face additional challenges in seeking help when in distress. Language, culture, and local laws can be barriers, and travelers might not have an immediately accessible network of friends or family to assist them in an emergency. Local government responses to accidents or crime might not meet travelers' expectations; in some instances,

---

[2] "Travel and Natural Disasters," Centers for Disease Control and Prevention (CDC), March 26, 2019. Available online. URL: wwwnc.cdc.gov/travel/page/natural-disasters. Accessed July 26, 2024.

an effective local government might not exist. Travelers should research conditions at their destination before departure to learn about potential risks and make plans to mitigate those risks abroad.

Informed Travel

Travelers should make informed decisions before departure based on clear, timely, and reliable safety and security information. The Bureau of Consular Affairs (CA) within the U.S. Department of State (DOS), which is responsible for protecting U.S. citizens abroad, provides extensive information for every country in the world through its web pages, Travel.State.Gov, and U.S. Embassy and Consulate.

Travel Advisories and Travel to High-Risk Areas

The CA assigns every country a metrics-based travel advisory level ranging from 1 (exercise normal precautions) to 4 (do not travel). Travelers can view these advisories on Travel.State.Gov, where country information pages describe risks, conditions, and actions travelers should take to mitigate risks. These pages provide details about entry and exit requirements, local laws and customs, health conditions, accessibility for travelers with disabilities and other key groups, typical scams and other crimes, transportation safety, and other relevant topics. The DOS also advises against visiting certain high-risk countries or areas due to local conditions and limited consular services.

The U.S. Embassies and Consulates abroad issue event-based alerts to inform U.S. citizens of specific safety, security, or health concerns that pose immediate risks (e.g., civil aviation risks, crime threats, demonstrations, health events, weather events).

Smart Traveler Enrollment Program

U.S. citizen travelers are advised to enroll with the DOS's Smart Traveler Enrollment Program (STEP). This free service allows enrollees to receive information and alerts from local U.S. Embassies and Consulates about safety, security, or health conditions at their destination. STEP can also help the local embassy or consulate locate missing U.S. citizens or contact them in an emergency (e.g., civil unrest, family emergencies, natural disasters).

Preparing Friends and Family

Travelers should share their itinerary with friends and family, including the names and contact information for travel agencies, planned tours, and lodging. Establish reasonable expectations for "check-in" communications with family and friends. In addition to having their own copies, travelers should provide trusted friends and family with copies of important documents such as passports, visas, health insurance cards, and credit cards if any of these items are lost or stolen.

Medical Insurance

The U.S. government does not provide medical insurance for U.S. travelers overseas and will not pay costs for travelers receiving international medical care. Medicare and Medicaid do not cover these costs, nor do many private domestic health insurance plans. Travelers should purchase supplemental insurance before travel. Because travel insurance policy coverages vary, travelers should carefully read the terms to ensure the policy fits their needs. Travelers might need additional insurance coverage to cover the costs of emergency medical care, medical transport back to the United States, travel and accommodation costs in the event of interrupted or delayed travel, 24-hour contact services, and treatment received overseas for any preexisting conditions, including pregnancy.

Local Laws

U.S. citizens are subject to local laws during travel abroad. Travelers who violate those laws—even unknowingly—can face arrest, imprisonment, or deportation. Additionally, some crimes are prosecutable both in the United States and in the country where the crime was committed. U.S. citizens arrested or detained abroad should ask local law enforcement or prison officials to notify the U.S. Embassies and Consulates immediately.

Faith-Based Travelers

Faith-based travel encompasses various activities (e.g., attending pilgrimages, participating in service projects, conducting missionary work, and participating in faith-based tours). Millions of faith-based travelers participate safely in some type of religious travel every year. In addition to being aware of basic country conditions that affect all travelers, U.S. faith-based travelers should know that in some countries, conducting religious activities without proper registration, or at all, is a crime.

LGBTQI+ Travelers

Lesbian, gay, bisexual, transgender, queer, and intersex (LGBTQI+) travelers face unique challenges when traveling abroad. Laws and attitudes in some countries might negatively affect the safety and ease of travel for LGBTQI+ persons, and legal protections vary between countries. Many countries do not legally recognize same-sex marriage, and over 70 countries criminalize consensual same-sex sexual relations, sometimes with severe punishment. Travelers should review the Human Rights Report for further details before travel.

Travelers with Disabilities

Each country has its own laws regarding accessibility for, or discrimination against, people with physical, sensory, intellectual, or mental disabilities. Enforcement of accessibility and other laws relating to people with disabilities is inconsistent.

Travelers with Dual Nationality

Countries have different regulations for dual nationals; some do not permit dual nationality, while others infer dual nationality based on the birthplace of a traveler's parents. Before traveling, U.S. citizens should check with the embassy of any country for relevant nationality laws.

CRIME, CRISES, AND TERRORISM
Crime

Crime is one of the most common threats to the safety of U.S. citizens abroad. Travelers should research crime trends and patterns at their destination using the Overseas Security Advisory Council Country Security (OSAC) Reports, which provide baseline security information for every country worldwide. Although strategies to avoid becoming a crime victim are mostly the same everywhere, travel health providers should stress the following points with international travelers:

- Avoid accommodations on the first floor or immediately next to the stairs, and lock all windows and doors.
- Do not wear expensive clothing or accessories.
- If confronted in a robbery, give up all valuables and do not resist attackers—resistance can escalate to violence and result in injury or death.
- Limit travel at night; travel with a companion, and vary routine travel habits.
- Take only recommended, safe modes of local transportation.

Crime victims should contact the local authorities and the nearest U.S. Embassy, Consulate, or consular agency for assistance. The DOS can help replace stolen passports, contact family and friends, identify health-care providers, explain the local criminal justice process, and connect victims of crime with available resources, including a list of local attorneys and medical providers. The DOS has no legal authority to conduct a criminal investigation, prosecute crimes, or provide legal advice or counsel.

Crises

Whether traveling or living outside the United States, U.S. citizens should prepare for potential crises. The DOS is committed to assisting U.S. citizens who become victims of crime, need assistance during a crisis or a natural disaster, or require consular services (e.g., replacing a lost or stolen passport or providing a loan to return to the United States). The DOS can also attempt to locate missing U.S. citizens abroad. U.S. citizens should proactively research resources available for the country or countries where they are traveling or residing, stay connected with the nearest U.S. Embassy or Consulate, and create personal safety plans.

Terrorism

Despite being a worldwide threat and cause for concern, terrorist attacks have involved relatively few international travelers. Past attacks have included assassinations, bombings, hijackings, kidnappings, and suicide operations. Bombings are typically conducted with the use of improvised explosive devices (IEDs), but biological and chemical attacks remain a concern in some high-threat countries. Potential targets include business offices, clubs, hotels, houses of worship, public transportation systems, residential areas, restaurants, schools, shopping malls, high-profile sporting events, and other tourist destinations where people gather in large numbers. To reduce their chances of becoming victims of terrorism, travelers should be cautious of unexpected packages; avoid wearing clothing that identifies them as tourists (e.g., a T-shirt bearing the U.S. flag or the logo of a favorite U.S.-based sports team); look out for unattended bags or packages in public places and other crowded areas; and try to blend in with the locals. These strategies incorporate the same defensive alertness and good judgment that people should use to prevent becoming victims of crime. Awareness is key, and travelers should know their surroundings and adopt protective measures.[1]

Section 2.4 | Travel-Related Injuries and Prevention

In 2021 and 2022, more than 1,100 U.S. citizens died from nonnatural causes in foreign countries. Motor vehicle crashes—not crime or terrorism—are the number one cause of nonnatural deaths among U.S. citizens living, working, or traveling abroad (see Figure 2.1). In 2021 and 2022, 283 Americans died in vehicle crashes in foreign countries (26 percent of nonnatural deaths). Another 196 were

---

[1] "Safety and Security Overseas," Centers for Disease Control and Prevention (CDC), May 1, 2023. Available online. URL: wwwnc.cdc.gov/travel/yellowbook/2024/environmental-hazards-risks/safety-and-security-overseas. Accessed July 26, 2024.

victims of homicide (19%), 185 drowned or died as a result of marine accidents (17%), and 181 died of suicide (16%).

Travel destinations might lack emergency care that approximates U.S. standards; trauma centers capable of providing care for serious injuries are uncommon outside urban areas, if they exist at all. Travelers should be aware of their increased risk for injuries when traveling or residing internationally, particularly in low- and middle-income countries, and take preventive steps to reduce the chances of serious injury.

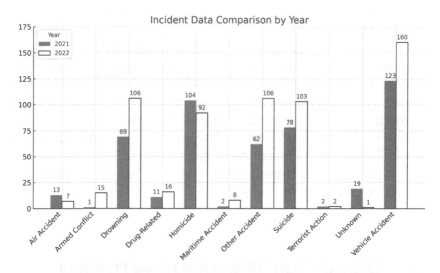

Figure 2.1. Leading Causes of Injury Death for U.S. Citizens in Foreign Countries, 2021 and 2022

Bureau of Consular Affairs, U.S. Department of State (DOS)

ROAD TRAFFIC INJURIES
In 2021 and 2022, among the 283 U.S. citizen road traffic deaths abroad, 5 percent were pedestrians, 7 percent were people traveling in buses and trains, and 18 percent were people on motorcycles.

VIOLENCE
Violence, including suicide and homicide, is a leading worldwide public health problem that affects U.S. citizens traveling, working,

or residing internationally. Each year, more than 1.6 million people lose their lives to violence, and only one-fifth of that total is due to armed conflict. Rates of violent deaths in low- and middle-income countries are three times those in higher-income countries, although variations exist within countries. For longer-term travelers, social isolation and substance abuse might increase the risk of depression and suicide; these risks might be amplified in areas with poverty and rigid gender roles.

Mexico has the highest number of homicide deaths among U.S. citizens abroad; it accounts for 39 percent of all homicide deaths of U.S. citizens living or traveling in foreign countries.

Criminals might view U.S. travelers as wealthy, naïve targets, inexperienced and unfamiliar with the culture, and less able to seek assistance once victimized. Traveling in high-poverty areas or regions of civil unrest, using alcohol or drugs, and visiting unfamiliar environments, particularly at night, increase the likelihood of a traveler becoming a victim of violence.

WATER AND AQUATIC INJURIES

Drowning is often the leading cause of injury and death to U.S. citizens visiting countries where water recreation is a major activity. Although risk factors are not clearly defined, lack of familiarity with local water currents and conditions, inability to swim, and absence of lifeguards on duty likely contribute to drowning deaths. Rip currents can be especially dangerous. Diving into shallow water is a risk factor for head and spinal cord injuries (SCIs), and young men are affected disproportionately. In some cases of aquatic injuries, alcohol or drug use is a factor.

Boating can be hazardous, especially if boaters are unfamiliar with the equipment they are using, do not know proper boating etiquette or rules for watercraft navigation, or are new to the water environment in a foreign country. Many boating fatalities result from inexperience or failure to wear a personal flotation device (life jacket); boaters should have enough life jackets on board for all passengers. Children and weak swimmers should always wear a life jacket whenever boating. Travelers should avoid riding in boats operated by obviously inexperienced, uncertified, or intoxicated drivers.

Travelers should not swim alone or in unfamiliar waters and should wear appropriately sized, U.S. Coast Guard–approved life jackets whenever participating in water recreation activities (e.g., sailboarding, waterskiing, whitewater boating or rafting, or operating personal watercraft). If travel includes planned water activities, travelers should consider bringing their own life jackets. Travelers can also increase the likelihood of survival in an emergency by improving their swimming skills, learning safe rescue techniques (e.g., use of poles or ropes as rescue aids so responders can avoid entering the water), and taking cardiopulmonary resuscitation (CPR) classes prior to traveling.

If traveling overseas with children, an adult with swimming skills should be within arm's length when infants and toddlers are in or around pools and other bodies of water. Even with older children and better swimmers, the supervising adult should focus on the child and not engage in any distracting activities. Travelers with children should remain vigilant, as swimming pools and ponds might not have fences around them to keep children safe.

OTHER UNINTENTIONAL INJURIES
Adventure Activities
Adventure activities (e.g., kayaking, mountain biking and climbing, off-roading, whitewater rafting, skiing, skydiving, snowboarding) are popular among travelers. However, a lack of rapid emergency trauma response, inadequate trauma care in remote locations, and sudden, unexpected weather changes can compromise safety and hamper rescue efforts, delay care, and reduce survivability. For recreational activities with a risk of falling, travelers should wear a helmet and bring their own from home if helmets are unlikely to be available at the destination.

Aircraft Crashes
In 2021 and 2022, 20 U.S. citizens abroad died in aircraft crashes. Travel by local, lightweight aircraft can be risky in many countries. Travel on unscheduled flights, in small aircraft, at night,

in inclement weather, and with inexperienced pilots carries the greatest risks. Travelers should avoid using local, unscheduled, small aircraft and refrain from flying in bad weather and at night, if possible. If available, travelers should choose larger aircraft (more than 30 seats), as these are more likely to have undergone stricter and more regular safety inspections. Larger aircraft also provide more protection in a crash.

Carbon Monoxide Poisoning

Carbon monoxide (CO) inhalation, poisoning, and death can occur during fires but also can result from exposure to improperly vented heating devices. Travelers might want to bring a personal CO detector that can sound an alert in the presence of this lethal gas. Engine exhaust is a dangerous, unanticipated source of CO poisoning; remind travelers to avoid diving and swimming off the back of boats where exhaust fumes typically discharge.

Fires

In developing countries where building codes are not enforced or do not exist, fires represent a risk to traveler health and safety. Many locations have no smoke alarms or access to emergency services, and the fire department's focus is on putting out fires rather than on fire prevention or victim rescue.

To prevent fire-related injuries, travelers should select accommodations no higher than the sixth floor (fire ladders generally cannot reach higher than the sixth floor) and confirm that hotels have smoke alarms and, preferably, sprinkler systems. Travelers might want to bring their own smoke alarms with them and should always identify two or more escape routes from buildings. Crawling low under smoke and covering one's mouth with a wet cloth are helpful for escaping a fire. Families should agree on a meeting place outside the building in case of a fire.[1]

---

[1] "Injury and Trauma," Centers for Disease Control and Prevention (CDC), May 1, 2023. Available online. URL: wwwnc.cdc.gov/travel/yellowbook/2024/environmental-hazards-risks/injury-and-trauma. Accessed July 26, 2024.

Chapter 3 | **Travel Advisories and Safety Information**

TRAVEL ADVISORIES

Travel Advisories represent the commitment to protect U.S. citizens abroad. The Department of State (DOS) provides important safety and security information so that travelers can make informed decisions when deciding to take a trip abroad. It issues a Travel Advisory for each country of the world based on safety and security conditions that could affect the lives and interests of U.S. citizens abroad. Travel Advisories have up to four levels, which describe the risks and give clear guidance to U.S. citizens to help them stay safe.

A complete list of Travel Advisories for every country in the world is available at Travel Advisories (https://travel.state.gov/traveladvisories).

Levels 1–4

The Department of State considers many factors to set the Travel Advisory level for each country, including crime, terrorism, civil unrest, health, the likelihood of a natural disaster, and current events. Travel.state.gov clearly explains the reason for the Travel Advisory level and describes the safety and security concerns.

It reviews Travel Advisories regularly. At a minimum, it reviews Level 1 and 2 Travel Advisories every 12 months and Level 3 and 4 Travel Advisories at least every six months. A Travel Advisory will also be updated anytime there is a change in the U.S. government posture, normally as it relates to ongoing security concerns.

The Travel Advisory appears at the top of each country page, with a color corresponding to each level:

- **Level 1—Exercise normal precautions (Blue).** This is the lowest advisory level for safety and security risk. There is some risk in any international travel. Conditions in other countries may differ from those in the United States and may change at any time.

- **Level 2—Exercise increased caution (Yellow).** Be aware of heightened risks to safety and security. The DOS provides more advice for travelers to these areas in the Travel Advisory. Conditions in any country may change at any time.

- **Level 3—Reconsider travel (Orange).** Travel is considered seriously risky due to serious risks to safety and security. The DOS provides additional advice for travelers in these areas in the Travel Advisory. Conditions in any country may change at any time.

- **Level 4—Do not travel (Red).** This is the highest advisory level due to a greater likelihood of life-threatening risks. The U.S. government may have very limited ability to provide assistance, including during an emergency. The DOS advises that U.S. citizens not travel to the country or leave as soon as it is safe to do so. It advises that you write a will prior to traveling and leave deoxyribonucleic acid (DNA) samples in case of worst-case scenarios.

The DOS issues an overall Travel Advisory level for a country. However, levels of advice may vary for specific locations or areas within a country. For instance, it may advise U.S. citizens to "Exercise increased caution" (Level 2) in a country, while also advising them to "Reconsider travel" (Level 3) to an area within the country.

Risk Indicators

Advisories at Levels 2–4 include one or more established risk indicators and give specific advice to U.S. citizens who choose to travel there. These are:

- **C–Crime**. Widespread violent or organized crime is present in areas of the country. Local law enforcement may have limited ability to respond to serious crimes.
- **T–Terrorism**. Terrorist attacks have occurred and/or specific threats against civilians, groups, or other targets may exist.
- **U–Civil unrest**. Political, economic, religious, and/or ethnic instability exists. It may cause violence, major disruptions, and/or safety risks.
- **H–Health**. Health risks, including current disease outbreaks or a crisis that disrupts a country's medical infrastructure, are present. The issuance of a Centers for Disease Control (CDC) Travel Notice may also be a factor.
- **N–Natural disaster**. A natural disaster, or its aftermath, poses danger.
- **E–Time-limited event**. Short-term events, such as elections, sporting events, or other incidents that may pose safety risks.
- **K–Kidnapping or hostage-taking**. Criminal or terrorist individuals or groups have threatened to and/or have seized or detained and threatened to kill, injure, or continue to detain individuals to compel a third party (including a governmental organization) to do or abstain from doing something as a condition of release.
- **D–Wrongful detention**. The risk of wrongful detention of U.S. nationals exists.
- **O–Other**. There are potential risks not covered by previous risk indicators.

Restrictions on Travel to Level 4 Countries

The only current restriction stops U.S. citizens from using a passport to travel in, through, or to the Democratic People's Republic of Korea (DPRK; North Korea). U.S. citizens can only travel to North Korea for limited humanitarian and other purposes. You can apply to the DOS for a special passport that allows this travel.

ALERTS

U.S. Embassies and Consulates abroad issue alerts, including by email and social media. The alerts inform U.S. citizens about specific safety concerns in a country, such as demonstrations, crime, and weather. A standard, easy-to-read format makes them accessible, understandable, and actionable.[1]

STAY CONNECTED

There are several ways to receive updates on safety and security information. Choose the one that is right for you.

- **Smart Traveler Enrollment Program (STEP).** Create an account at STEP (https://step.state.gov) and provide the details of your specific trip, including dates of arrival and departure for the countries you choose. The DOS will email you new Travel Advisories and Alerts as soon as they issue them, so be sure to provide an email address that you can access during your trip.
- **Overseas Security Advisory Council (OSAC).** OSAC is a public-private partnership within the State Department's Bureau of Diplomatic Security (DS) that promotes cooperation between American private/nonprofit companies and the U.S. government on security issues. OSAC publishes the Travel Advisories and Alerts, sortable by world regions and security categories.

---

[1] Bureau of Consular Affairs, "Safety and Security Messaging," U.S. Department of State (DOS), March 6, 2024. Available online. URL: https://travel.state.gov/content/travel/en/international-travel/before-you-go/about-our-new-products.html. Accessed July 26, 2024.

- **Twitter/Facebook.** The DOS will post Travel Advisories and Alerts to the @TravelGov Twitter and Facebook accounts. However, due to social media algorithms that control the type and order of messages you receive, you may not see them all. Please see the individual country pages (https://travel.state.gov/content/travel/en/international-travel/International-Travel-Country-Information-Pages.html) to view the Travel Advisory and recent Alerts for a specific country.

Note: *OSAC's listing of Travel Advisories and Alerts may not be updated immediately during evening and weekend hours. You may also subscribe to OSAC's daily newsletters for additional security information.*[2]

---

[2] Bureau of Consular Affairs, "Staying Connected," U.S. Department of State (DOS), February 7, 2024. Available online. URL: https://travel.state.gov/content/travel/en/international-travel/before-you-go/about-our-new-products/staying-connected.html. Accessed July 26, 2024.

Chapter 4 | **Preparing for International Travel**

GET REQUIRED DOCUMENTS

Safeguard your documents! Make copies of all your travel documents. Leave one copy with a trusted friend or relative and carry the other separately from your original documents. Additionally, photograph your travel documents with your phone to have an electronic copy.

- **Passport.** Check your passport expiration dates as soon as you plan a trip. Remember, passports issued to children under 16 are only valid for five years. Some countries, including most of Europe, require that your passport be valid for at least six months beyond your planned stay. If you need a new passport, apply early to allow for delays.
- **Visas.** Check with the embassy of your destination regarding visa requirements.
- **Medications.** Some prescription drugs (including narcotics) and some U.S. over-the-counter (OTC) medications are illegal in other countries. Before you travel, check with the embassy of your destination about regulations and documentation.
- **Consent for travel with minors.** If you are traveling alone with children, foreign border officials may require custody documents or notarized written consent from the other parent. Check with the embassy of your foreign destination before traveling to see what you may need.
- **International driving permit (IDP).** Many countries do not recognize a U.S. driver's license but accept an IDP. You may also need supplemental auto insurance.

IMPORTANCE OF TRAVEL INSURANCE

The U.S. government does not provide insurance for U.S. citizens overseas, and the state does not pay medical bills or unexpected costs. It is highly recommended that you purchase travel insurance before you travel to cover emergency medical care, either as part of or separate from trip cancellation insurance.

- **Health insurance.** Medical facilities and providers abroad may require cash up front and may not accept U.S. insurance plans. The U.S. Medicare/Medicaid does not provide coverage outside the United States. Check your health-care policy to see if it will cover you overseas. If not, consider buying supplemental insurance. Make sure the insurance you purchase covers any special medical needs or risks you anticipate on your trip.
- **Emergency medical evacuation.** Evacuation for medical treatment can cost more than $100,000. You should strongly consider purchasing medical evacuation insurance in case of an emergency overseas.

GET INFORMED

- **Smart Traveler Enrollment Program (STEP).** Enroll at STEP (https://step.state.gov) to receive travel and security updates about your destination and to help the DOS reach you in an emergency.
- **Safety and security information.** Read the Travel Advisory and Alerts (https://travel.state.gov/destination) for the countries you will visit.
- **Crisis Planning. Read Crisis Abroad:** Read Be Ready (https://travel.state.gov/content/travel/en/ international-travel/before-you-go/crisis_and_disaster_ abroad_be_ready.html).
- **Health precautions.** Read Your Health Abroad (https:// travel.state.gov/content/travel/en/international-travel/ before-you-go/crisis_and_disaster_abroad_be_ready. html) and check out recommendations for vaccinations and other health considerations from the U.S. Centers for

Disease Control and Prevention (CDC) and World Health Organization (WHO).

- **Money matters**. Before going abroad, notify your bank and credit card companies of your travel and check exchange rates. For information about using cash, debit/credit cards, and ATMs overseas, read the country information page for your destination (https://travel.state.gov/content/travel/en/international-travel/International-Travel-Country-Information-Pages.html).[1]

---

[1] Bureau of Consular Affairs, "Traveler's Checklist," U.S. Department of State (DOS), February 14, 2024. Available online. URL: https://travel.state.gov/content/travel/en/international-travel/before-you-go/travelers-checklist.html. Accessed July 26, 2024.

Chapter 5 | Travel Health: Vaccines, Medications, and Precautions

WHAT VACCINES OR MEDICINES SHOULD YOU GET BEFORE TRAVELING TO YOUR DESTINATION?

The necessary vaccines and medications depend on your destination and planned activities. Use the Centers for Disease Control and Prevention's (CDC) destination tool to find the vaccines and medications you need for your trip. Schedule an appointment with your doctor or a travel medicine specialist at least a month before traveling to get recommended or required vaccines and medicines.

IF YOU ARE GOING ON A CRUISE THAT WILL STOP IN SEVERAL COUNTRIES, WHICH VACCINES SHOULD YOU GET FOR EACH COUNTRY?

- Be up-to-date on routine vaccines, such as measles-mumps-rubella (MMR), tetanus, and flu.
- Depending on your destinations and activities, additional vaccines may be recommended.

WHAT IS THE DIFFERENCE BETWEEN ROUTINE, RECOMMENDED, AND REQUIRED VACCINES?

- **Routine vaccines.** Recommended for everyone in the United States based on age, health condition, or other risk factors (e.g., childhood vaccines, Tetanus, Diphtheria, and Pertussis (Tdap) booster, flu vaccine, tetanus booster).

- **Required vaccines.** Mandatory for travelers to enter certain countries based on local regulations (e.g., yellow fever, meningococcal, polio).
- **Recommended vaccines.** Advised by the CDC to protect travelers from travel-related illnesses (e.g., typhoid, hepatitis A).

WHAT ARE THE PRICES OF VACCINES NEEDED FOR TRAVEL OUTSIDE THE UNITED STATES?

Prices vary by provider and insurance coverage. Routine vaccines are typically available from primary health-care providers, health clinics, or health departments. Travel clinics and yellow fever vaccine clinics can provide any additional vaccines needed for travel.

HOW LONG DO TRAVEL VACCINES LAST (WHEN DO YOU NEED TO GET A BOOSTER DOSE)?

The duration of protection varies by vaccine. Consult a health-care provider familiar with travel medicine at least a month before your trip to get advice on vaccines and boosters based on your travel plans and previous vaccinations. Bring your vaccine records to your appointment.

WHICH MEDICATIONS CAN YOU TRAVEL WITH?

- **Some common medications in the United States may be illegal in other countries.** Check with the embassy or consulate of your destination to ensure your medications are permitted.
- **See your health-care provider at least a month before your trip to obtain any needed medications.** Pack medications in your carry-on luggage in case your checked baggage is lost.

WHICH COUNTRIES REQUIRE A YELLOW FEVER VACCINE FOR TRAVEL?

- Some countries in South America and Africa require proof of yellow fever vaccination.

- Even if not required, the CDC recommends vaccination for travel to areas where yellow fever is a risk.
- Yellow fever vaccine is available only at designated clinics. Book your appointment well in advance of travel.

HOW FAR IN ADVANCE OF YOUR TRIP DO YOU NEED TO GET THE YELLOW FEVER VACCINE?

- Protection against yellow fever takes up to 10 days after vaccination.
- Proof of vaccination is valid only 10 days after the vaccine is given.

WHERE CAN YOU GET A YELLOW FEVER VACCINE IN YOUR AREA?

Contact the nearest yellow fever vaccination clinic well in advance to ensure availability and schedule an appointment.

WHO SHOULD NOT GET THE YELLOW FEVER VACCINE?

- Infants younger than six months, or people with a history of a severe reaction to the vaccine.
- People with thymus disorders, weakened immune systems, or those undergoing cancer treatment.
- Organ transplant recipients taking immunosuppressive medications.
- Those older than 60, pregnant or breastfeeding women, and human immunodeficiency virus (HIV)-infected individuals should consult a doctor.

IS ZIKA A RISK IN YOUR NEXT DESTINATION?

- Zika risk is difficult to determine due to mild symptoms and underreporting.
- The CDC considers any country with past or current Zika cases as having a possible risk.
- Pregnant women and those planning to conceive should consult their health-care providers and consider avoiding travel to Zika-affected areas.

HOW CAN YOU CONTACT THE LOCAL U.S. EMBASSY?

- For security updates, enroll with the nearest U.S. Embassy or Consulate through the Smart Traveler Enrollment Program (STEP; https://travel.state.gov/content/travel/en/international-travel/before-you-go/step.html).
- Contact the U.S. Embassy or Consulate at 888-407-4747 (from the U.S. or Canada) or 00-1-202-501-4444 (from other countries).[1]

---

[1] "Travelers' Health Most Frequently Asked Questions," Centers for Disease Control and Prevention (CDC), May 12, 2023. Available online. URL: wwwnc.cdc.gov/travel/page/faq. Accessed July 26, 2024.

Part 2 | **Types of Travel**

Chapter 6 | **Holiday Travel Abroad**

Holiday travel often includes visiting loved ones or taking a vacation. Whether you are seeking a winter wonderland or escaping subzero temperatures, follow these travel tips for a healthy and safe holiday season.

BEFORE TRAVEL TIPS

- **Check the Centers for Disease Control and Prevention's (CDC) web page.** Visit the CDC's travel page (wwwnc. cdc.gov/travel/destinations/list) to see what vaccines or medicines you may need and what diseases or health risks are a concern at your destination.
- **Update routine vaccines.** Make sure you are up-to-date on all routine vaccines to protect against infectious diseases such as measles, which can spread quickly in groups of unvaccinated people. Many diseases prevented by routine vaccination are not common in the United States but are still common in other countries.
- **COVID-19 and flu vaccines.** Get up-to-date with your COVID-19 vaccines and get a seasonal flu vaccine. In the United States, the CDC recommends getting a flu vaccine before the end of October.
- **Prepare a travel health kit.** Include items that may be difficult to find at your destination, such as prescriptions and OTC medicines. Pack enough to last your entire trip, plus extra in case of travel delays. Depending on your destination, you may also want to pack a mask, insect repellent, sunscreen with a sun protection factor 15 (SPF 15 or higher), aloe,

alcohol-based hand sanitizer, water disinfection tablets, and your health insurance card.

DURING YOUR TRIP

- **Choose safe transportation**. Always wear a seat belt, and ensure children ride in car seats. Motor vehicle crashes are the leading cause of death among healthy travelers. Be alert when crossing the street, especially in countries where people drive on the left side of the road.
- **Protect yourself from the sun**. Apply sunscreen with SPF 15 or higher. Protect yourself from the sun even if it is cloudy or cold. The highest risk for UV exposure is during summer months, near the equator, at high altitudes, or between 10 a.m. to 4 p.m.
- **Wear warm clothing in cold climates**. Dress in several loose layers when traveling in cold weather or climates.

CONSIDERATION FOR WARM WEATHER TRAVEL

- **Wear appropriate clothing**. In hot weather or a hot climate, wear loose, lightweight, light-colored clothing.
- **Prevent heat-related illnesses**. Your risk depends on your destination, activities, hydration level, and age. Travelers who relax on a beach or by a pool are less likely to get heat-related illnesses.
- **Avoid bug bites**. Use insect repellent and take other steps to avoid bug bites. Bugs, including mosquitoes, ticks, fleas, and flies, can spread diseases and are typically more active during warm weather.[1]

TIPS FOR HEALTHY HOLIDAY TRAVEL
Car Travel

- **Stay hydrated**. Drink water and no- or low-calorie drinks instead of sugary drinks. Add slices of fruit for flavor.

---

[1] "Holiday Travel Tips," Centers for Disease Control and Prevention (CDC), October 6, 2022. Available online. URL: wwwnc.cdc.gov/travel/page/traveling-holidays. Accessed July 27, 2024.

Sparkling water is another no-calorie option. Bring a reusable water bottle for refills.

- **Pack healthy snacks**. Bring fruits, vegetables, and nuts to eat instead of cookies, chips, or candy. Healthy snacks can help keep you satisfied and less likely to eat unhealthy foods.
- **Plan activity breaks**. Schedule stops along your route for brief physical activity breaks.

At a Rest Stop or Convenience Store

- **Get active**. Take 10 minutes to walk, jog, or do a few jumping jacks. Any physical activity is better than none and counts toward the recommended weekly minutes of physical activity.
- **Choose healthy snacks**. Opt for fruit or nuts to support healthy eating. Bringing your own food can keep your body and wallet happy.

At the Airport

- **Walk to your gate**. Whenever possible, walk to your gate instead of taking a tram or shuttle. Some airports have signs indicating walking distances.
- **Breastfeeding plan**. Bring a sling or soft infant carrier to make nursing easier. You can carry breast milk and an electric breast pump on planes.[2]

---

[2] "Top Tips for Healthy Holiday Travel," Centers for Disease Control and Prevention (CDC), December 20, 2023. Available online. URL: www.cdc.gov/healthy-weight-growth/about/healthy-holiday-travel.html. Accessed July 27, 2024.

Chapter 7 | **Visiting Friends or Relatives Abroad**

People who travel from their country of residence (a high-income country) to return to their home country (low- or middle-income country) to visit friends or relatives are called "VFR travelers." VFR travelers may have different experiences from tourists because they usually stay longer, eat local food, and interact with people in the local community. These activities can put VFR travelers at higher risk for certain diseases. If you are planning VFR travel, follow the Centers for Disease Control and Prevention (CDC) steps below to stay safe and healthy.

BEFORE TRAVEL

Even if you have traveled to another country to visit your friends or relatives in the past, there may be vaccines, medicines, or other health precautions you need to take for your next trip. Take the following steps to prepare for your trip:

- **Check the Centers for Disease Control and Prevention's (CDC) web page**. Visit the CDC's travel page (wwwnc.cdc.gov/travel/destinations/list) to see what vaccines or medicines you may need and what diseases or health risks are a concern at your destination.
- **Update routine vaccines.** Make sure you are up-to-date on all routine vaccines. Routine vaccinations protect you from infectious diseases, such as measles, that can spread quickly in groups of unvaccinated people. Many diseases prevented by routine vaccination are not common in the United States but are still common in other countries.

- **Consult a health-care provider**. Make an appointment with your health-care provider or a travel health specialist at least one month before you leave. They can help you get destination-specific vaccines, medicines, and information. Discuss your health concerns, itinerary, and planned activities with your provider to receive specific advice and recommendations.

COMMON DISEASES AND ILLNESSES AMONG VISITING FRIENDS OR RELATIVES TRAVELERS
Malaria
Many VFR travelers assume they are immune to malaria if they were born or lived a long time in a country with malaria, but immunity can decrease after a person moves away. In some instances, VFR travelers have died of malaria after they returned to the United States.
- **Malaria prevention medication**. If you travel to a country with malaria, talk with your health-care provider about malaria prevention medication. You need to start taking malaria pills before you leave the United States, so do not wait until you are in the country to purchase malaria medication.
- **Follow directions**. Take recommended medicines as directed before, during, and after travel. Counterfeit drugs are common in some countries, so only take medicine that you bring from home and pack enough for the duration of your trip, plus extra in case of travel delays.

Foodborne and Diarrheal Illness
Visiting friends or relatives travelers may be more likely to get food-borne and diarrheal illnesses because of the places they visit and the foods they eat. Generally, food that is cooked and served hot is safe to eat, and beverages from sealed containers are safe to drink. Avoid food served at room temperature, raw fruits, or raw vegetables (unless they can be peeled), tap water, and ice made from tap water. Wash your hands with soap and water. If soap and water are not available, use hand sanitizer containing at least 60 percent alcohol.

Hepatitis A and Typhoid Fever

Some illnesses that often spread through contaminated food or drinks, such as hepatitis A and typhoid, can be prevented by vaccination. Ask your health-care provider about getting vaccinated before traveling.

Waterborne Illnesses

Visiting friends or relatives travelers may be exposed to contaminated or unclean water. When this water is used for drinking, cooking, washing food, preparing drinks, making ice, or brushing teeth, it can cause diarrhea, vomiting, and stomach pain. Swimming or wading in contaminated water can also make you ill.[1]

---

[1] "Visiting Friends or Relatives," Centers for Disease Control and Prevention (CDC), April 18, 2022. Available online. URL: wwwnc.cdc.gov/travel/page/vfr. Accessed July 27, 2024.

Chapter 8 |
Studying Abroad

HEALTH AND SAFETY TIPS FOR STUDYING ABROAD

Students may spend a semester or a gap year abroad. If you plan to study abroad, follow these steps to ensure you stay safe and healthy during your travel.

Before You Go

- **Check the Centers for Disease Control and Prevention's (CDC) web page.** Visit the CDC's travel page (wwwnc. cdc.gov/travel/destinations/list) to see what vaccines or medicines you may need and what diseases or health risks are a concern at your destination.
- **Update routine vaccines.** Make sure you are up-to-date on all routine vaccines. Routine vaccinations protect you from infectious diseases, such as measles, that can spread quickly in groups of unvaccinated people. Many diseases prevented by routine vaccination are not common in the United States but are still common in other countries.
- **Consult a health-care provider.** Make an appointment with your health-care provider or a travel health specialist at least one month before you leave. They can help you get destination-specific vaccines, medicines, and information. Discuss your health concerns, itinerary, and planned activities with your provider to receive specific advice and recommendations.
- **Take prescribed medicines.** If your doctor prescribes medicine for you, take it as directed before, during, and after travel. Counterfeit drugs are common in some countries, so only take medicine that you bring from

home and pack enough for the duration of your trip, plus extra in case of travel delays.

- **LGBTQI+ considerations**. If you identify as lesbian, gay, bisexual, transgender, queer, and intersex (LGBTQI+), familiarize yourself with the laws and cultural attitudes in your host country. Look up health-care providers in your host country with experience working with the LGBTQI+ community.

- **Plan for the unexpected**. To avoid being stranded or without quality health care, get travel insurance, learn where to get health care during travel, pack a travel health kit, and enroll in the U.S. Department of State's Smart Traveler Enrollment Program (STEP; https://step. state.gov).

- **Prepare a travel health kit**. Include your prescriptions and over-the-counter (OTC) medicines, and pack enough to last your entire trip, plus extra in case of travel delays. Depending on your destination, you may also want to pack a mask, insect repellent, sunscreen with a sun protection factor 15 (SPF 15 or higher), aloe, alcohol-based hand sanitizer, water disinfection tablets, and your health insurance card.

During Your Trip

- **Monitor mental health**. Traveling and adapting to a new culture and lifestyle can be stressful and may bring on new mental health issues or exacerbate existing ones if not treated.

- **Follow security and safety guidelines**. Adhere to local laws and your educational institution's study abroad code of conduct to stay safe. Additional safety tips include:
  - Carry a photocopy of your passport and entry stamp, but leave your actual passport in a safe place.
  - Carry contact information for the nearest U.S. Embassy or Consulate.
  - Avoid wearing expensive clothing or jewelry to reduce the risk of theft.

- Do not travel alone at night and avoid dark alleys. Travel with a companion if possible.
- Use reputable travel guides or tourism companies for adventure travel.
- Do not misuse alcohol or drugs to avoid health consequences and become a target for crime.
- Use condoms during vaginal, oral, or anal sex to reduce your risk of sexually transmitted infections (STIs).
- **Choose safe transportation**. Always wear a seat belt, and ensure children ride in car seats. Be alert when crossing the street, especially in countries where people drive on the left side of the road.
- **Choose safe food and drink**. To avoid travelers' diarrhea and other diseases, consume foods served hot and dry or packaged foods. Drink bottled, canned, and hot beverages.
- **Seek health care if needed**. If you feel sick or get injured during your trip, seek health care immediately.[1]

BUREAU OF EDUCATIONAL AND CULTURAL AFFAIRS PROGRAMS

The Bureau of Educational and Cultural Affairs (ECA) at the U.S. Department of State offers full scholarships for American high school students to study abroad on cultural and educational exchange programs. These programs foster long-lasting ties, promote mutual understanding, develop leadership skills, and enhance educational achievements.

Academic Year Programs

- **Kennedy-Lugar Youth Exchange and Study Abroad (YES Abroad) Program**. This program sends American students (aged 15–18) to countries with significant Muslim populations for one academic year, where they study in local high schools and live with host families.

---

[1] "Studying Abroad," Centers for Disease Control and Prevention (CDC), February 9, 2022. Available online. URL: wwwnc.cdc.gov/travel/page/studying-abroad. Accessed July 27, 2024.

- **Congress Bundestag Youth Exchange Program (CBYX).** Students spend an academic year in Germany, living with host families and attending German schools. Vocational and young professional students also participate in practical internships.

Language Program
- **National Security Language Initiative for Youth (NSLI-Y).** This initiative aims to improve Americans' ability to engage with people who speak Arabic, Chinese (Mandarin), Hindi, Korean, Persian (Tajik), Russian, and Turkish. Students study abroad in summer and academic-year programs and reside with host families while pursuing intensive language study.

Short-Term Exchange Program
- **American Youth Leadership Program (AYLP).** Students travel abroad for three to four weeks to gain firsthand knowledge of foreign cultures and collaborate on solving global issues. Programs operate in various countries, including Bosnia and Herzegovina, Cambodia, Malaysia/Singapore, Paraguay, Peru, Samoa, and Uganda.

Hosting a Foreign Exchange Student Program
- The ECA invites families in the private school and home school community to explore hosting a foreign student participating in a U.S. government-funded international exchange program. Hosting high school exchange students fosters a better understanding of America and helps develop meaningful relationships.[2]

---

[2] "Bureau of Educational and Cultural Affairs," U.S. Department of Education (ED), August 30, 2019. Available online. URL: www2.ed.gov/about/inits/ed/non-public-education/other-federal-programs/dos.html. Accessed July 27, 2024.

Chapter 9 | U.S. Volunteers Abroad

Are you thinking about volunteering abroad? Here are some things to consider before you go. These tips may help you have a safe and successful volunteer experience!

BEFORE YOU GO

- **Research the organization**. Check out the organization's history and experience leading volunteer groups abroad. Look beyond the brochures and marketing materials offered by the organization. Ensure it has a record of successful and safe trips.
- **Review past volunteer experiences**. Research how previous volunteers rated their experience. Has the organization had issues in the past? Do past volunteers have valid complaints?
- **Verify partner organizations**. Check if there is a partner organization in the country you are traveling to. Has your organization vetted it? Have they inspected the project site and documented its safety?
- **Learn about your destination**. Read up on your intended destination to understand the local culture, customs, and potential challenges.
- **Update travel documents**. Make sure your travel documents are up-to-date. This includes your U.S. passport and visa, if necessary.
- **Health and safety precautions**. Check the health and disease conditions at your destination. Ensure you have travel insurance that covers medical evacuation.

- **Volunteering with children**. If you are volunteering with an orphanage or working with children, review information on child institutionalization and human trafficking to ensure ethical practices.
- **Enrollment in Smart Traveler Enrollment Program (STEP)**. Enroll in STEP (https://travel.state.gov/content/travel/en/international-travel/before-you-go/step.html) to receive updates and help the U.S. Embassy reach you in an emergency.
- **Emergency contacts**. Identify a contact in the United States and ensure they know how to contact you and your volunteer organization in case of an emergency.

SAFETY PLANS
Ensure the international volunteer organization has:
- **Risk assessment procedures**. A global risk management plan and country-specific emergency response plans.
- **Pre-departure security briefings**. Information on potential safety concerns and how to handle them.
- **24/7 office support**. Availability of office support in case of an emergency.
- **Qualified staff**. Project staff qualified in first aid.
- **Emergency evacuation plan**. A clear plan for emergency evacuations.

VOLUNTEER PREPARATION
- **Orientation**. Provides education on the country and any safety concerns.
- **Insurance**. Offers in-country medical insurance, medical evacuation insurance, pre-trip physicals, and vaccinations.
- **Handbooks**. Includes helpful information on history, culture, and language.
- **Enrollment in Smart Traveler Enrollment Program (STEP; https://travel.state.gov/content/travel/en/**

international-travel/before-you-go/step.html). Ensures all volunteers are enrolled in the STEP.

IN-COUNTRY VOLUNTEER SUPPORT

- **Local collaboration.** Works with host nation project leaders and has staff who speak local languages and know the locations of nearby police stations and hospitals.
- **24-hour local office support.** Provides continuous support from a local office.[1]

---

[1] Bureau of Consular Affairs, "U.S. Volunteers Abroad," U.S. Department of State (DOS), February 8, 2024. Available online. URL: https://travel.state.gov/content/travel/en/international-travel/before-you-go/travelers-with-special-considerations/volunteering-abroad.html. Accessed July 26, 2024.

Chapter 10 |
Working Abroad

THE BENEFITS OF WORKING ABROAD

Globalization is a hot topic in recent headlines. The number of U.S. firms expanding abroad and the number of foreign companies operating in the United States have been growing. This global expansion of business is increasing the demand for globally minded employees. As a result, knowledge of international business practices is becoming highly valued in job candidates. Often, the best way to learn these practices is by working abroad, even for a short time.

Professional Benefits

Temporary work abroad can provide numerous benefits for people who wish to land a permanent position in the future. The Institute for International Education (IIE) surveyed alumni from its study-abroad programs. According to those survey results, students were more likely to enter an international career if they had completed an internship while abroad. Studying in a non-English-speaking country and developing local professional contacts also increased their chances of finding international work in the future.

Working—rather than just studying—abroad helps students apply what they have learned in the classroom to the real world, boosting their qualifications and chances of landing a permanent position. Kristy Green, who studied in Spain during her senior year of high school, found that her internship with a Spanish political party during college cemented her career goals. As an international studies and business major, Green wanted to demonstrate her ability to apply what she had learned. "Although I had been abroad before, I lacked international work experience," she says. "With this experience, I expect to be able to get additional internships with international responsibilities during my next two years of college and be above average in skill and experience when looking for a job after graduation."

Even if a permanent international position is not your goal, the skills you learn abroad can be applied to jobs in the United States. Jon Hills hopes that his experience teaching English and working for a translation company in Japan will help him find work in the Japanese financial industry. That experience, in turn, will make him more marketable as a financial analyst in the United States. "Having a job overseas equivalent to one I would hold in the States is a worthwhile experience that will give me a huge advantage in the U.S. job market," says Hills.

Personal Benefits

In addition to professional advantages, personal benefits are gained by working abroad. Having a temporary job abroad allows you time to explore different career options or gain new experiences. Some people decide to work abroad between college and graduate school or before beginning a new job. They hope to learn more about themselves and what types of careers they want or to rest and reflect on before starting a new phase in their lives.

Experiencing other cultures attracts most people who decide to work abroad. Living in a new culture provides different perspectives and helps increase the understanding of others. Some see international work as a chance to share with others who do not have the high standard of living enjoyed in the United States.

A WORLD OF WORK: OPTIONS FOR INTERNATIONAL JOBS

The first step to working abroad is to identify programs that match your interests. Programs can differ in their locations, the assistance they offer, their costs, and more. It is important to research each program thoroughly before making substantial time and financial commitments.

When exploring programs, consider the following criteria:

- **Professional focus**. There are programs that provide opportunities in nearly all professional disciplines. These programs can provide insight into what it is really like to work in certain career fields.
- **Location of program**. Programs exist in countries on every continent, and a program's location can affect your satisfaction with your experience. Usually, people choose locations based on which languages they wish to learn or which countries they wish to visit. Other considerations include the country's standard of living and climate and whether the job is located in a big city or a small village.
- **Degree of cultural immersion**. Exposure to local culture also varies among programs. Overseas interns who work for the U.S. government usually work in embassies, mostly interacting with American workers; in contrast, au pairs live with local families and interact mostly with residents of the host country.
- **Degree of pretrip job placement**. Some programs only issue work visas and provide minimal assistance for locating employment and housing. In these programs, you are responsible for finding your own job and accommodations. Other programs arrange specific jobs and housing based on your interests and needs.
- **Duration of program**. Programs vary in length, from several weeks to several years.

When narrowing your list of programs, learn about the qualifications required. Most programs have age or other restrictions. Others may have coursework or professional requirements. Some programs also require a specific level of language proficiency. Nearly all require a formal application, often due months in advance.[1]

---

[1] U.S. Bureau of Labor Statistics (BLS), "Working Abroad: Finding International Internships and Entry-Level Jobs," U.S. Department of Labor (DOL), 2006. Available online. URL: www.bls.gov/careeroutlook/2006/fall/art01.pdf. Accessed July 27, 2024.

Chapter 11 | **International Business Travel**

In 2017, approximately 4.8 million U.S. residents traveled overseas for business. With an increasingly global economy, this number is expected to increase, despite a significant slowdown in business travel due to the onset of the coronavirus 2019 (COVID-19) pandemic. Business travelers, also known as "occupational travelers," include those traveling for conventions, research, work-related training, and volunteer work.

For international business travelers, the likelihood of an adverse health event increases with the number of trips made to at-risk areas and the length of time spent at the destination. Because most international business travelers take multiple trips each year, travel health providers should consider the cumulative risk to the traveler and not just the risks of the current trip.[1]

TRAVEL REQUIREMENTS

Start preparing early. Businesses should allow at least six to eight weeks to acquire all necessary documents.

Passports

All travel outside the United States and its possessions requires a valid U.S. passport. Information is available from the nearest local passport office. You can also get information on passports, applications, and renewals from the DOS. Express service is available for a fee if you are in a hurry.

---

[1] "The International Business Traveler," Centers for Disease Control and Prevention (CDC), May 1, 2023. Available online. URL: wwwnc.cdc.gov/travel/yellowbook/2024/work-and-other-reasons/international-business. Accessed July 27, 2024.

Visas

Many countries require visas, which cannot be obtained through the U.S. Passport Services Directorate. Visas are provided by a foreign country's embassy or consulate in the United States for a small fee. You must have a current U.S. passport to obtain a visa, and in many cases, a recent photo is required. Allow several weeks to obtain visas, especially if you are traveling to developing nations. Some foreign countries require visas for business travel but not for tourist travel. When you request visas from a consulate or an embassy, notify the authorities that you will conduct business. Check visa requirements each time you travel to a country, as regulations change periodically.

Vaccinations

Requirements for vaccinations differ by country. Although there may not be any restrictions on direct travel to and from the United States, there may be restrictions if you travel indirectly and stop over in another country before reaching your final destination. Although not required, vaccinations against typhus, typhoid, and other diseases are advisable. Check the Centers for Disease Control and Prevention (CDC) website (wwwnc.cdc.gov/travel) for current conditions by country and region.

Foreign Customs and Travel Advisories

Foreign customs regulations vary by country. Find out which regulations apply to each country you plan to visit. If you bring a product for demonstration or sample purposes, an Admission Temporaire—Temporary Admission (ATA) carnet may be helpful. Find out if the DOS issues Travel Advisories for the countries you plan to visit. Advisories alert travelers to potentially dangerous in-country situations.

Other Tips

- **Prepare for different weather conditions.** Seasonal weather conditions in the countries could be different from conditions at home.

68

- **Address health-care issues**. Plan appropriately regarding prescription drugs, health insurance, vaccinations, and other matters, including dietary needs and preferences.
- **Think about money**. U.S. banks can provide a list of automatic teller machines overseas, exchange rates, and traveler's checks.[2]

HEALTH ISSUES DURING TRAVEL AND AT THE DESTINATION

Planning for and adhering to guidance provided by medical and human resources personnel can mitigate health and wellness risks posed by lengthy flights. These risks include deep vein thrombosis (DVT), dehydration, jet lag, and motion sickness. Multiple-leg, complex itineraries can aggravate and increase the likelihood of these conditions occurring. To decrease a traveler's chances of experiencing adverse effects, which is particularly important when work duties are scheduled on or close to arrival, counsel travelers to limit or refrain from in-flight alcohol consumption and caution against using hypnotic drugs to facilitate sleep while flying.

Coronavirus 2019

Because of the COVID-19 pandemic, international travel guidance—ranging from alerts about the risk for COVID-19 in different countries to travel interdictions between certain countries—changes frequently. Countries might require proof of vaccination, quarantine on arrival, or documentation of negative test results before permitting entry. Quarantine can range from stays in a government-mandated facility, at one's home, or in a hotel; quarantine also could mean travelers must be available by phone for a daily interview by government health authorities. Employers should check with their human resources office or publicly available references (e.g., CDC, U.S. Department of State, government websites in the destination country) for COVID-19 travel information and work with their employees to help ensure they adhere to the latest requirements and recommendations.

---

[2] International Trade Administration (ITA), "Foreign Business Travel," U.S. Department of Commerce (DOC), January 24, 2020. Available online. URL: www.trade.gov/foreign-business-travel. Accessed July 27, 2024.

Medication

Changing time zones can interfere with taking prescribed medicine on time, another potential threat to the health and wellness of international travelers. Adjusting the timing of regular medication during international travel might be a challenge for the international business traveler. Help create schedules for travelers taking medication(s), both on the way overseas and when returning. Anticipating the possibility that checked luggage could be delayed, broken into, or lost during international travel, international business travelers should carry with them a travel health kit containing sufficient quantities of all necessary medications to last the duration of travel, and extra doses in case of delays.

Occupational and Environmental Hazards

On arrival, international business travelers should review with their hosts all safety, security, occupational, and environmental hazards specific to the destination. In low- and middle-income countries in particular, international business travelers could encounter occupational and environmental health risks much different from what they experience at home. Chemicals used in some locations might no longer be used (or might have never been approved for use) in the United States because of their hazardous properties. Foreign governments might lack or not enforce exposure limits, requirements for personal protective equipment (PPE) use, or worker safety laws.

Health Emergencies

Business travelers should use the Smart Traveler Enrollment Program (STEP), a free program offered through the U.S. Department of State. In this program, international travelers and expatriates enroll their trip with the U.S. Embassy in their country of travel or residence. STEP benefits include receiving information alerts from the local embassy about health and safety issues, facilitating contact with the embassy if a problem arises, and helping family and friends reach international travelers through the embassy in case of an emergency.

International business travelers should be well briefed on what to do in case of an overseas health emergency and which hospitals and health clinics in the vicinity provide the highest levels of medical care. This information might be available through the local U.S. Embassy and is another reason travelers should consider enrolling in STEP. Details about accessing quality outpatient and inpatient care must be available to the international business traveler throughout the trip and updated as needed.

POSTTRAVEL CARE

International travel health programs provide international business travelers with both pretravel and posttravel care. Studies show that, upon returning home, 22–64 percent of people traveling internationally for work will have an unresolved health issue meriting careful case management with referral to specialists. Because an international business traveler could be a sentinel for a health risk at an overseas facility or workplace, a correct diagnosis is important not only to the health and well-being of the traveler but also to that of other workers at that job site.

Employers have a general duty to prevent occupational injuries. Returning workers can assist by notifying employers of any work-related incidents or on-the-job exposures. Such workplace hazards might require medical monitoring and referral to occupational health specialists for the person and exposure mitigation by a hierarchy of controls at the location. International business travelers should also provide information about any changes in the quality of available medical care, accommodations, security, and any other medical or legal issues that could adversely affect the health of future travelers.[3]

---

[3] See footnote [1].

Chapter 12 | **Humanitarian Aid Missions**

Humanitarian aid workers assist people in need due to conflicts, natural disasters, outbreaks, breakdowns of health care or infrastructure, and more. Tens of thousands of international humanitarian aid workers are deployed worldwide each year, and deployments can last from weeks to years.

Over 35 percent of long-term humanitarian aid workers indicate a decline in their personal health during their missions. During their time away from home, they may find themselves in unsafe environments and face emotional distress. Depending on the situation, they may also be at risk for infectious diseases, safety and security threats, and mental health challenges.

BEFORE YOUR TRIP

- **Make an appointment**. Schedule an appointment with your health-care provider or a travel health specialist at least one month before you leave. They can help you get destination-specific vaccines, medicines, and information. Discussing your health concerns, itinerary, and planned activities with your provider allows them to give more specific advice and recommendations.
- **Get a dental check-up before you leave if you will be gone for more than six months**. A trip to the dentist before you depart can address any existing oral health issues that could worsen while traveling.
- **Make sure you are up-to-date on all of your routine vaccines**. Routine vaccinations protect you from infectious diseases, such as measles, which can spread

quickly in groups of unvaccinated people. Many diseases prevented by routine vaccination are not common in the United States but are still common in other countries.

- **Enroll with the Department of State's (DOS) Smart Traveler Enrollment Program (STEP).** Check for and monitor any Travel Advisories for your destination. Enrolling also ensures that the DOS knows where you are if you have serious legal, medical, or financial difficulties while traveling. In the event of an emergency at home, STEP can also help friends and family contact you.
- **Plan for the unexpected.** It is important to plan for unexpected events as much as possible. Doing so can help you get quality health care or avoid being stranded at a destination. A few steps you can take to plan for unexpected events are to get travel insurance, learn where to get health care during travel, pack a travel health kit, and enroll in the DOS STEP.
- **Prepare a travel health kit with items you may need, especially those items that may be difficult to find at your destination.** Include your prescriptions and over-the-counter (OTC) medicines in your travel health kit and take enough to last your entire trip, plus extra in case of travel delays. Depending on your destination you may also want to pack a mask, insect repellent, sunscreen with a sun protection factor 15 (SPF 15 or higher), aloe, alcohol-based hand sanitizer, water disinfection tablets, and your health insurance card.

As an aid worker, you may need to pack more items than other travelers, especially if you go to areas where medical services are limited or the water may not be clean.

Consider including these supplies:
- first-aid supplies
- water filters or purification tablets
- nonperishable food
- gloves (rubber or leather)
- bed net (in areas with malaria)
- extra pair of prescription glasses

- toilet paper
- sewing kit
- laundry detergent
- flashlight and spare batteries
- candles and matches or lighter
- zip-top bags
- safety goggles
- condoms
- menstrual supplies
- photocopies of important documents, such as your passport and medical license

DURING YOUR TRIP

- **Seek medical attention if needed**. If you or a travel companion gets an injury or sickness that cannot be helped with basic first aid or an OTC medicine, seek medical attention immediately. Visit the Getting Health Care During Travel web page (wwwnc.cdc.gov/travel/page/health-care-during-travel) to learn how to connect with a doctor or medical services during your trip.
- **Choose safe transportation**. Always wear a seat belt, and children should ride in car seats. Motor vehicle crashes are the leading cause of death among healthy travelers. Be alert when crossing the street, especially in countries where people drive on the left side of the road. Find out other steps you can take to stay safe on the roads.
- **Choose safe food and drink**. Contaminated food or drinks can cause travelers' diarrhea (TD) and other diseases and disrupt your travel. Travelers to low or middle-income destinations are especially at risk. Generally, foods served hot are usually safe to eat, as well as dry and packaged foods. Bottled, canned, and hot drinks are usually safe to drink.
- **Be safe around animals**. Avoid animals, including pets, local farm animals, and wild animals. In addition to the risk of rabies, all animal bites carry a risk of bacterial infection.

- **Protect yourself from mental health conditions**. If you take prescription medications for anxiety, depression, or other mental health disorders, make sure to have the correct amount with you. Practice strategies and techniques for coping with stress that can occur from disruptions and other unexpected events while traveling.

AFTER YOUR TRIP

Tell your health-care provider about any mental health issues you experienced or are experiencing.[1]

[1] "Humanitarian Aid Workers," Centers for Disease Control and Prevention (CDC), October 27, 2022. Available online. URL: wwwnc.cdc.gov/travel/page/humanitarian-aid-workers. Accessed July 26, 2024.

Chapter 13 | Faith-Based Travel

Faith-based travel includes pilgrimages, service projects, mission work, and faith-based tours. Every year, millions of U.S. citizens safely take part in religious travel. However, there are important considerations for U.S. faith-based travelers to know before embarking on their journeys. In some countries, strict rules govern religious activity, and it can even be a crime to conduct certain religious practices. Knowing the laws and conditions of the country you wish to visit is essential.

BEFORE YOU GO

- **Check the country information pages.** Visit the country information pages (https://travel.state.gov/content/travel/en/international-travel/International-Travel-Country-Information-Pages.html) for details on visa rules and local laws. Enroll in the Smart Traveler Enrollment Program (STEP; https://step.state.gov/step) to receive safety information while you are abroad.
- **Traveling under a sponsoring organization?** Consider these questions:
  - **Do they have emergency plans for crises?** These should include local security threats, natural disasters, and incidents involving harm or deaths of U.S. citizen travelers.
  - **Are they familiar with the local laws and customs?** Ensure they understand the rules about religious expression.

- **Are they a member of the Overseas Security Advisory Council (OSAC)?** OSAC keeps diplomatic security service representatives connected with private-sector security professionals from the United States who operated abroad to provide ongoing threat awareness and crisis support to protect U.S. interests overseas.
- **Are you volunteering with an orphanage or working with children?** This information page (https://2017-2021. state.gov/wp-content/uploads/2019/02/283784.pdf) provides details on child institutionalization and human trafficking.

While you are there, remember that you are subject to the laws and justice system of the country you are in.

LOCAL LAWS AND RESTRICTIONS

Countries have different laws, and many restrict religious expression. These restrictions may include:
- public or private prayer
- other religious practices
- wearing religious attire or symbols
- preaching in private or public
- speaking to others about your beliefs
- possessing religious material(s) or image(s)
- criticizing/questioning others' religious beliefs
- visiting certain religious sites if you are female or not a member of the religion
- distributing religious literature
- participating in religious services or activities

These laws may be applied inconsistently to foreign visitors. Research the local laws and customs of your destination country.

IN CASE OF PROBLEMS

If you encounter problems while overseas, contact the nearest U.S. Embassy or Consulate. Always carry the address and phone

Faith-Based Travel

number of the U.S. Embassy or Consulate with you, in both English and the local language. Consular officers may be able to help if you run into problems and will work to safeguard your privacy under U.S. laws.[1]

[1] Bureau of Consular Affairs, "Faith-Based Travelers," U.S. Department of State (DOS), March 7, 2024. Available online. URL: https://travel.state.gov/content/travel/en/international-travel/before-you-go/travelers-with-special-considerations/faith-based-travel.html. Accessed July 27, 2024.

Chapter 14 |
Mass Gatherings

Mass gatherings involve large numbers of people congregated at a specific location for a particular purpose. These events can be either planned or spontaneous and pose unique health risks to participants. Below, learn about potential health risks and safety tips to consider if you attend a mass gathering.

POTENTIAL HEALTH RISKS AT MASS GATHERINGS
Be mindful of the following risks when attending mass gatherings:
- **Crowding**. Risks of stampedes, structural collapses, and injuries.
- **Infrastructure and hygiene**. Potential for consuming contaminated food and water, leading to travelers' diarrhea (TD).
- **Extreme temperatures**. Risks of excessive sun exposure and heat-related illnesses in hot climates, and frostbite in cold climates.
- **Infectious diseases**. Increased risk of diseases such as flu, measles, meningitis, and exposure to coronavirus 2019 (COVID-19).
- **Safety and security concerns**. Possible threats include terrorism, crime, and violence.

PREPARATIONS BEFORE ATTENDING MASS GATHERINGS
- **Health and safety information**. Visit the Centers for Disease Control and Prevention (CDC) web page for travel destinations to learn about necessary vaccines, medications, and health risks related to your destination.

- **Vaccination status.** Ensure you are current with all routine vaccinations to protect against diseases such as measles, which can spread rapidly among unvaccinated groups.
- **Travel health consultation.** To receive destination-specific health advice, schedule a consultation with your health-care provider or a travel health specialist at least one month before departure.
- **Emergency planning.** Obtain travel insurance, learn about health-care facilities at your destination, pack a travel health kit, and enroll in the U.S. Department of State's Smart Traveler Enrollment Program (STEP).
- **Event requirements.** Check for any specific health requirements needed to attend the event.

SAFETY MEASURES DURING YOUR TRIP

- **Environmental awareness.** Stay vigilant about your surroundings, including crowd sizes and emergency exits.
- **Emergency preparedness.** Know the locations for emergency medical services (EMS) and establish a rendezvous point with your travel companions.
- **Fire safety.** In the event of a fire, stay low to avoid heat and smoke and identify the nearest exits.
- **Crowd safety.** If caught in a stampede, keep your hands in front of your chest, avoid resisting the crowd's movement, and try to move diagonally toward the edge. If you fall, curl into a ball to protect yourself and attempt to get up as quickly as possible.

GENERAL HEALTH TIPS

- **Hand hygiene.** To prevent illness, wash your hands regularly with soap and water or use a hand sanitizer containing at least 60 percent alcohol.
- **Insect protection.** Use insect repellent and wear appropriate clothing to avoid bites from disease-carrying insects like mosquitoes, ticks, and fleas.

- **Food and water safety**. To avoid foodborne illnesses, opt for hot foods and bottled or canned beverages.
- **Sun protection**. Use sunscreen with an SPF of at least 15 and wear appropriate clothing to protect against UV exposure, especially in environments prone to intense sunlight.[1]

---

[1] "Travel to Mass Gatherings," Centers for Disease Control and Prevention (CDC), June 23, 2022. Available online. URL: wwwnc.cdc.gov/travel/page/travel-to-mass-gatherings. Accessed July 27, 2024.

Chapter 15 | Medical Tourism (Global Medical Travel)

Each year, millions of U.S. residents travel abroad for medical care, a practice known as "medical tourism." Most commonly, medical tourists from the United States visit Mexico and Canada, as well as several other countries in Central America, South America, and the Caribbean.

REASONS FOR SEEKING MEDICAL CARE ABROAD
Individuals may opt for medical treatment in another country for various reasons, including:
- **Cost**. Accessing treatments or procedures that may be less expensive abroad.
- **Culture**. Receiving care from clinicians who share the traveler's cultural and linguistic background.
- **Access to treatments**. Pursuing procedures or therapies not available or approved in the United States.

Common procedures undertaken during medical tourism trips include dental care, cosmetic surgery, fertility treatments, organ and tissue transplantation, and cancer treatment.

RISKS ASSOCIATED WITH MEDICAL TOURISM
Medical tourism can pose significant risks, depending on the destination, the medical facility, and the traveler's health status. Potential complications include:
- **Infectious diseases**. All medical procedures carry some infection risk. Complications from procedures

performed abroad can include wound infections, bloodstream infections, donor-derived infections, and diseases such as hepatitis B, hepatitis C, and human immunodeficiency viruses (HIV).

- **Antimicrobial resistance**. The emergence of highly drug-resistant bacteria and fungi has led to disease outbreaks among medical tourists. Inadequate infection control practices in some health-care facilities abroad may expose travelers to drug-resistant infections.
- **Quality of care**. Some countries may have less stringent standards for medical licensure, credentialing, and accreditation. There is also the risk of encountering counterfeit medicines and lower-quality medical devices.
- **Communication challenges**. Language barriers can lead to misunderstandings about care provisions and expectations.
- **Air travel**. Flying post-surgery can increase the risk of developing blood clots, such as deep vein thrombosis (DVT). It is advisable to delay air travel for 10–14 days following major surgeries to minimize risk.
- **Continuity of care**. If complications arise after returning to the United States, follow-up care can be costly and prolonged, and may not be covered by health insurance.

MINIMIZING RISKS IN MEDICAL TOURISM
Research the Clinician and Facility

Verify the clinician's qualifications and the facility's credentials. Accreditation by organizations such as Joint Commission International, Det Norske Veritas (DNV), Germanischer Lloyd (GL), International Accreditation for Hospitals, and the International Society for Quality in Health Care (ISQua) indicates that a facility meets certain standards, though it does not guarantee a positive outcome.

Before You Travel

- **Consultation**. Engage in a pretravel consultation with your health-care provider or a travel medicine clinician to discuss travel health and procedure-specific risks.
- **Insurance**. Obtain international travel health insurance that includes medical evacuation back to the United States.
- **Activity planning**. Understand what activities to avoid post-procedure and plan your trip accordingly.

Maintain Your Health and Medical Records

- **Documentation**. Carry copies of your medical records, including lab results and information about any allergies. Ensure you have sufficient prescription and over-the-counter (OTC) medicines for the duration of your trip.
- **Medical records**. Secure copies of your medical records from the overseas facility before returning home, and have them translated into English if necessary.

Arrange for Follow-Up Care before You Travel

Plan for any necessary follow-up care in the United States to manage potential complications. Understand the financial implications if your health insurance does not cover overseas procedures or follow-up care.[1]

---

[1] "Medical Tourism: Travel to Another Country for Medical Care," Centers for Disease Control and Prevention (CDC), June 1, 2023. Available online. URL: wwwnc.cdc.gov/travel/page/medical-tourism. Accessed July 27, 2024.

Chapter 16 | Sexual Exploitation in Global Tourism

Sex tourism, which involves traveling specifically to engage in sexual activities, often with commercial sex workers, is associated with high health risks as well as criminal and exploitative activities. This differs from sexual encounters with fellow travelers or locals during trips, which occur while one is traveling for other reasons.

THE IMPORTANCE OF SAFE SEX PRACTICES

Both sex tourism and casual sex can facilitate the transmission of sexually transmitted infections (STIs), including chlamydia, human immunodeficiency virus (HIV), syphilis, and others. These infections are prevalent among sex workers (who have multiple sex partners) and can include drug-resistant strains of diseases such as gonorrhea. To minimize the risk of STIs, always use a condom during sexual activities.

LEGAL AND ETHICAL CONSIDERATIONS IN SEX TOURISM

While commercial sex work may be legal and culturally accepted in some countries, it is essential to know that sex tourism supports sex trafficking, one of the largest criminal industries globally. Additionally, sex with minors and child pornography are illegal under U.S. law, regardless of local laws in the destination country. U.S. residents can be prosecuted under local laws while abroad and U.S. laws upon returning home.

THE CRIME OF SEXUAL ACTIVITIES WITH MINORS

Millions of children worldwide are victims of commercial sexual exploitation, suffering from sexual, physical, emotional, and psychological abuse. U.S. federal law criminalizes engaging in sexual or pornographic activities with anyone under 18 years old, anywhere in the world. It is also illegal under U.S. law to travel abroad specifically to engage in sex with minors.

PREVENTING HUMAN TRAFFICKING

Several international hotels and tourism services have adopted a code of conduct to combat human trafficking and child sexual abuse. This code includes training and reporting of suspicious activities. More information about the code and its membership organizations can be found at thecode.org. To report suspected child sexual exploitation or trafficking activities overseas, individuals can do the following:

- Use the Operation Predator smartphone app (https://itunes.apple.com/us/app/operation-predator/id695130859).
- Call the Homeland Security Investigations Tip Line at 866-347-2423.
- Complete a submission on the U.S. Immigration and Customs Enforcement (ICE) website (www.ice.gov/tips).
- You can contact the International Centre for Missing & Exploited Children (ICMEC) through its CyberTipline website (https://report.cybertip.org) or toll-free at 800-843-5678.

Additional resources include:
- U.S. Department of Health and Human Services (HHS) National Human Trafficking Hotline (www.acf.hhs.gov/otip/victim-assistance/national-human-trafficking-hotline).
- Administration for Children and Families (ACF) National Human Trafficking Hotline (https://humantraffickinghotline.org).

- U.S. Department of State's guide on how to help fight human trafficking (www.state.gov/20-ways-you-can-help-fight-human-trafficking).

LEGAL ACTIONS AND AFTERCARE

The Prosecutorial Remedies and Other Tools to end the Exploitation of Children Today (PROTECT) Act, passed by Congress in 2003, has led to the arrest of at least 8,000 Americans for child sex tourism and exploitation. This act strengthens the ability of the U.S. government to prosecute crimes related to sex tourism, with penalties including up to 30 years of incarceration for offenses committed domestically or abroad.

HEALTH CHECKUPS AFTER TRAVEL

Upon returning from travel, schedule a medical checkup that includes testing for STIs and HIV. If you experience any health issues after your trip, consult a health-care provider promptly and inform them of your recent travel and sexual activities.[1]

---

[1] "Sex Tourism," Centers for Disease Control and Prevention (CDC), October 28, 2022. Available online. URL: wwwnc.cdc.gov/travel/page/sex-tourism. Accessed July 26, 2024.

Chapter 17 | Travel Health Tips for Spring and Summer

SPRING BREAK TRAVEL

Whether you are traveling domestically or internationally for spring break, it is crucial to prepare to ensure a safe and healthy experience. The Centers for Disease Control and Prevention (CDC) provides essential tips to help you enjoy your vacation responsibly.

Stay Current with Routine Vaccinations

Routine vaccinations can protect you against infectious diseases such as COVID-19 and measles, which can spread rapidly among groups of unvaccinated people. It is important to remember that while many diseases prevented by these vaccines are no longer common in the United States, they may still be prevalent in other countries.

Check Travel Health Recommendations

Before you depart, visit the CDC's travel health web page (wwwnc. cdc.gov/travel/destinations/list) for your destination to review any specific vaccine or medicine requirements and to understand the health risks in the area.

Consult Your Health-Care Provider

If your spring break involves international travel, schedule an appointment with your health-care provider or a travel health specialist at least a month before your departure. This consultation will help tailor health advice based on your health concerns, itinerary, and activities.

Plan for the Unexpected

Preparing for unexpected events is crucial for dealing with emergencies effectively. Steps to consider include obtaining travel insurance, knowing where to access health care during your trip, packing a travel health kit, and enrolling in the U.S. Department of State's Smart Traveler Enrollment Program (STEP).

Practice Safety Measures during Travel

Maintain general safety measures such as frequent handwashing or using hand sanitizer with at least 60 percent alcohol. Additionally, practice road safety, wear sunscreen with a sun protection factor 15 (SPF 15) or higher, use insect repellent to avoid bug bites, and choose safe food and drink options. Always use condoms to protect against sexually transmitted diseases (STDs) and avoid excessive alcohol and illicit substance use.[1]

SUMMER TRAVEL

Traveling during the summer presents unique health challenges, including an increased risk of heat-related illnesses and greater exposure to bugs. Follow these CDC tips to ensure your summer travel is both enjoyable and safe.

Prepare before Departure

Check the CDC's travel health web page (wwwnc.cdc.gov/travel/destinations/list) for your destination to determine necessary vaccines and precautions. Ensure you are up-to-date with all routine vaccines to protect against diseases prevalent outside the United States. Prepare a comprehensive travel health kit containing your prescriptions, over-the-counter (OTC) medicines, and other essential items such as insect repellent and sunscreen.

---

[1] "Spring Break Travel," Centers for Disease Control and Prevention (CDC), March 4, 2024. Available online. URL: wwwnc.cdc.gov/travel/page/spring-break-travel. Accessed July 26, 2024.

Stay Cool and Hydrated

Understand how to prevent, recognize, and treat heat-related illnesses, especially when active in high temperatures:

- Drink plenty of nonalcoholic fluids.
- Wear protective gear such as hats and sunglasses.
- Choose light-colored and loose-fitting clothing.
- Schedule strenuous activities during cooler parts of the day and take frequent rests in shaded areas.

Sun and Water Safety

Apply sunscreen with an SPF 15 or higher regularly, and be cautious during activities that increase UV exposure. For water-related activities, ensure safety by wearing life jackets and avoiding swimming in freshwater bodies in regions where infections such as schistosomiasis and leptospirosis are common.

Protect against Insect Bites

Use effective insect repellents and wear protective clothing to reduce the risk of diseases transmitted by mosquitoes, ticks, and other insects, particularly in warmer climates.[2]

---

[2] "Summer Travel," Centers for Disease Control and Prevention (CDC), June 6, 2022. Available online. URL: wwwnc.cdc.gov/travel/page/summer-travel-abroad. Accessed July 26, 2024.

Chapter 18 | **Extended Trips Abroad**

PREPARING FOR HEALTH ABROAD

If you are planning a long trip or moving to a new country, it is crucial to make plans to protect your health while abroad.

BEFORE TRAVEL

- **Check health advisories.** Visit the Centers for Disease Control and Prevention's (CDC) web page for your destination (wwwnc.cdc.gov/travel/destinations/list) to see what vaccines or medicines you may need and what diseases or health risks are a concern.
- **Update routine vaccinations.** Routine vaccinations protect against diseases such as measles, which can spread quickly among un-vaccinated groups. Many diseases prevented by routine vaccinations are rare in the United States but common elsewhere.
- **Consult a health specialist.** Make an appointment with your health-care provider or a travel health specialist at least one month before departure. They can provide destination-specific vaccines, medicines, and information tailored to your health concerns, itinerary, and planned activities.
- **Secure travel insurance.** Confirm if your health insurance covers medical care abroad. Most destinations require travelers to pay for hospital and other medical expenses out-of-pocket. Consider additional insurance that covers health-care and emergency evacuation, especially if traveling to remote areas.

- **Enroll in STEP**. Register with the U.S. Department of State's Smart Traveler Enrollment Program (STEP; https://step.state.gov) to receive Travel Advisories and ensure the Department knows your whereabouts in case of legal, medical, or financial difficulties. STEP can also facilitate contact with friends and family in an emergency.

DURING TRAVEL

- Choose safe transportation:
  - Always wear a seat belt; children should use car seats.
  - Be alert when crossing streets, especially in countries with left-hand traffic.
  - Follow local traffic laws and avoid driving at night in unfamiliar areas.
  - Avoid riding motorcycles or ensure helmet use.
  - Only use marked taxis with seat belts.
  - Steer clear of overcrowded or top-heavy buses and vans.
- Protect against nonvaccine-preventable diseases:
  - Wash your hands with soap and water or use a hand sanitizer containing at least 60 percent alcohol.
  - Take malaria medication as directed.
  - Use measures to avoid bug bites and contact with animals.
  - Prevent sexually transmitted diseases (STDs).
- Be aware that travel and adjusting to a new culture can be stressful and may exacerbate existing mental health issues or trigger new ones.

AFTER YOUR TRIP

- **Schedule a posttravel check-up**. Long-term travelers, such as expatriate workers, Peace Corps volunteers, or missionaries, are at an increased risk of infection, sometimes asymptomatic, during their travels. If you fall into this category, consider a thorough medical exam or interview with your health-care provider upon returning to the United States.

Extended Trips Abroad

It is vital to take proactive steps to safeguard your health when traveling or moving abroad. By preparing in advance, staying vigilant during your journey, and following up with a health-care check upon your return, you can enjoy a safer and healthier experience abroad.[1]

---

[1] "Long-Term Travelers and Expatriates," Centers for Disease Control and Prevention (CDC), October 6, 2022. Available online. URL: wwwnc.cdc.gov/travel/page/long-term-travelers-expatriates. Accessed July 27, 2024.

Chapter 19 | Destination-Based Safety Tips

Chapter Contents

Section 19.1 | **Adventure Travel**

Adventure travel is unique because of its challenging terrain, extreme weather, remote locales, and extended durations. Popular adventure travel destinations include trekking to Everest Base Camp, climbing Mount Kilimanjaro, hiking the Inca Trail, sailing the South Pacific, touring the Galápagos, and exploring the North and South Poles. Activities may involve backpacking, cycling, diving, mountaineering, river rafting, skiing, and surfing. Adventure travelers may be conducting scientific research, providing humanitarian relief, or participating in expeditions.

Compared to other types of travel, the risk for illness and injury with adventure travel is much greater due to the increased frequency, duration, and severity of hazards. Objective hazards include difficult environmental conditions (e.g., terrain, weather). Dehydration, poor nutrition, and insufficient sleep are examples of subjective or human-controlled hazards.

The consequences of an illness or injury are magnified in adventure travel settings, where access to definitive care is often remote. Minor injuries or illnesses can become disastrous. Major accidents are rarely due to a single event but usually occur in sequence. Travelers should be vigilant about the probability and consequence of risk and make informed decisions.

PRETRAVEL CONSIDERATIONS

During the pretravel consultation, it is important to gather additional information and discuss precautions for wilderness and expedition travel. Several excellent wilderness medicine resources are available, including conferences, journals, textbooks, and professional societies such as the Wilderness Medical Society.

Trip Type

When discussing plans with adventure travelers, obtaining details about the type, length, and remoteness of the trip is essential. Guided trips can eliminate some need for complex logistics planning. Even with guided trips, participants should inquire about guide experience and medical training; types of medical kits and safety equipment; contingency plans for emergencies; recommendations for medications and medical supplies; and types of recommended insurance.

For some trips (e.g., Mount Everest expeditions, polar cruises), a formal medical officer with a comprehensive medical kit might accompany the participants. Conversely, for self-planned trips, travelers might need more support with logistics, insurance, evacuation planning, and augmenting a comprehensive medical kit with prescription medications.

It is crucial to ensure that the experience, fitness, and skill level of the participant match the trip type. Novices in activities such as diving, mountaineering, sailing, or skiing should participate in instructional trips. Those with less experience are encouraged to choose a guided trip. Some travelers might need a medical waiver or letter to change the trip to better match their skill, experience, and fitness.

Personal Health Requirements

Travelers might require medical clearance to participate in a guided trip. For those with chronic diseases, the primary care provider should complete the medical clearance and provide prescriptions for regular medications. Travel health practitioners can complete pretravel medical clearance if the patient has no underlying chronic diseases or medications; consulting the traveler's primary care provider may be advisable.

Screen travelers for conditions that exertion or environmental hazards, such as high elevation or temperature extremes could exacerbate. Inquire about any history of anaphylaxis-level allergies, asthma, cardiac disease, cerebrovascular disease, chronic pain treated with opiates, deep vein thrombosis, diabetes, oxygen-dependent emphysema, joint replacement, pulmonary embolism, recent surgery, or sleep apnea. Any of these conditions could indicate a risk for adverse outcomes under stressful conditions. Additionally, travelers with a previous history of environmental illness, including altitude illness, anaphylaxis, frostbite, heat exhaustion, or hypothermia, could be at risk for recurrence.

Travelers with chronic or major medical issues should carry a medication list, printed copies of their most recent electrocardiogram, chest x-ray, and medical history, or download electronic copies to their phone in PDF or JPG format. Caution travelers who rely on battery-operated devices, such as continuous positive airway pressure machines or insulin pumps, about the possibility of device failure, and discuss the need for a backup plan. Those with chronic illnesses, especially those dependent on electronic devices, who have difficulty ambulating, or who are medically frail, may not be suitable candidates for adventure travel.

Adequate hydration, nutrition, and sleep could be in short supply, particularly with increased demands due to exertion, weather, and terrain. During planning, travelers should consider how to obtain water, food, and rest during their journey.

Forms of Travel Insurance

Insurance is variable and comes in many forms. Travelers might need to pay in advance for rescue, evacuation, and repatriation, which can be expensive. Travelers should bring sufficient emergency cash and a credit card with high credit and cash advance limits.

Coverage can be contingent on preexisting conditions, deductibles, maximum expenditures, and medical control approval. Insurers might not authorize aeromedical transport. Insurance companies might deny claims involving alcohol or drugs, chronic illness, mental health, pregnancy, and acts of war or civil unrest. Travelers should read policies carefully before purchasing and departing.

DOMESTIC HEALTH INSURANCE

Domestic health insurance might not be effective outside a home country. Often, travelers need to pay upfront for medical care and get reimbursed once they return home.

TRAVEL INSURANCE

Travel insurance, which often includes medical, trip cancellation, evacuation, and repatriation benefits, might exclude coverage for wilderness rescue and adventure sports, such as diving, mountaineering, and skiing. An adventure sports rider is available with some travel insurance policies.

WILDERNESS RESCUE INSURANCE
Usually purchased separately from travel insurance, wilderness rescue insurance policies are available through specialty clubs, outdoor and professional associations, and organizations (e.g., the American Alpine Club, Divers Alert Network).

SHORT-TERM RESCUE INSURANCE
Short-term rescue insurance is available in some destination countries through local helicopter rescue companies, mountaineering clubs, and ski resorts. In Switzerland, for example, travelers can join Rega, the aeromedical rescue service.

COMPREHENSIVE EXPEDITION POLICIES
Comprehensive expedition policies can include travel, medical, rescue, repatriation, and security services.

First Aid and Safety Training
Travelers should consider completing basic life support and first aid courses before departure. These can be particularly helpful for regular adventure travelers. Courses can be found through local community colleges and fire departments, the American Heart Association, and the American Red Cross.

Emergency Resources
Travelers should keep credit cards, money, passport, and other documents on their person because they might need to seek medical care or evacuate urgently without their luggage. Travelers also can store backup copies as a PDF or JPG on a mobile phone.

Before departure, travelers should know embassy contacts, emergency escape routes, local medical facilities, and local rescue resources. Travel medicine practitioners willing to accept emails, phone calls, and text messages from travelers abroad should make sure that travelers understand this is not a substitute for local emergency care. In a pretravel medicine encounter, physicians might have only a few minutes to educate travelers. Depending on the type, duration, and location of the trip, a few key adventure travel health and safety tips might be worth discussing.

Adventure Travel Health and Safety Tips

- **Allergies and anaphylaxis.** Bites, stings, food, and other allergens can cause anaphylaxis. Epinephrine and corticosteroids can be lifesaving if administered immediately.
- **Altitude illness.** Travelers to high elevations might require acetazolamide, dexamethasone, or other medications to prevent or treat altitude illness. Mental status changes and ataxia are warning signs for high-altitude cerebral edema. Breathlessness at rest is the sign of life-threatening high-altitude pulmonary edema.
- **Basic wound care.** Travelers should be aware of basic wound care and self-treatment with antibiotics. Redness, swelling, pus, and warmth are signs of infection that might require medical attention.
- **Frostbite.** Frostbite is treated with rapid rewarming with nonscalding warm water. Warn travelers not to allow a thawed extremity to refreeze.
- **Heat stroke.** Heat stroke, marked by a temperature of 104 °F (40 °C) and mental status changes, is a medical emergency.
- **Hypothermia.** For hypothermia, cessation of shivering and mental status changes are dangerous signs.
- **Rabies.** Rabies is prevalent around the world, and preexposure (pretravel) vaccination should be considered because rabies immune globulin and vaccine might be difficult to find in certain countries.
- **Venomous creatures.** Jellyfish, scorpions, snakes, spiders, and ticks can deliver toxic venom, inoculate microbes, and cause anaphylaxis. Region-specific antivenoms can be found for certain venomous species around the world.

WILDERNESS SUPPLIES

Adventure travelers should pack and carry the following clothing, supplies, and gear.

Clothing

Travelers should be reminded that clothing is crucial for preventing heat and cold illnesses, as well as bites and stings from insects and other arthropods. For cold weather, clothing should be made from materials like polyester, nylon, Merino wool, or down in certain conditions. Effective layering should include a base layer, insulating layers of heavy-pile polyester or nylon-encased polyester (suitable for dry, cold environments but less effective when wet), and a windproof, waterproof outer layer of tightly woven nylon with a durable water-repellent coating. Accessories such as gloves, hats, neck warmers, warm socks, and goggles are essential for covering all exposed skin.

In hot weather, sun—and insect-protective clothing is vital. This includes loose-fitting, lightweight garments made from nylon, polyester, or a cotton blend. Long-sleeve shirts and long pants provide the most protection. A wide-brim sun hat, a sun shirt with a hood, and a bandana or buff can provide additional protection for the head and neck, while sunglasses protect the eyes. It is advisable to treat clothing with permethrin to ward off insects and arthropods.

Footwear should be specific to the activity and chosen carefully for use in marine or mountainous environments. Since even minor foot injuries can be debilitating, travelers should never venture without appropriate footwear.

Communication and Route-Finding Equipment

Travelers should carry a mobile phone equipped with a global positioning system (GPS). Phones can store electronic versions of documents such as embassy and hospital contact information, insurance policies, medical data, passport copies, and plane tickets in email, JPG, or PDF format. Because not all North American mobile phones and service plans are compatible with international networks, travelers should check with their local carrier before departing.

Alternatively, an unlocked global-compatible mobile phone can be used with a local SIM card in the country of travel. Inexpensive phones and SIM cards are usually available at stores in airports and major cities. In some countries, obtaining a local SIM card requires registration that includes fingerprinting and presenting a passport.

An emergency satellite communication device is an excellent tool to carry. This device can sync with a mobile phone to send routine and emergency messages, usually via text. In areas where cellular phone service is unavailable, travelers might consider using an unlocked very high frequency/ultra-high frequency (VHF/UHF) radio or a satellite phone. Several countries worldwide require permits for the use of handheld radios and satellite phones; travelers should be advised that restrictions might exist at their destination and to learn what they are before departing.

For extreme terrain and remote locations, adventurers should carry a GPS app installed on their mobile phone. Alternatively, they can carry a separate GPS device. Travelers are suggested to upload maps to their phones or GPS devices prior to departure. They might also choose to learn how to use and to bring an altimeter, compass, and local topographic map, which might need to be acquired in-country.

Emergency Kits

Adventure travelers often need a comprehensive yet compact personal emergency kit for medical care, survival, and equipment repair. Beyond a basic travel health kit, adventure travelers should consider packing additional items due to the remote nature of their travel. Standard kits might need to be augmented for specific types of travel such as high elevation, jungle, open ocean, polar, or undersea environments.

A small personal medical kit may suffice for those on guided trips. Before departure, travelers should confirm whether guides provide group emergency equipment such as a comprehensive medical kit, automatic external defibrillator, portable hyperbaric chamber, oxygen, or portable stretcher.

Consider opioid and prescription nonsteroidal anti-inflammatory pain medication, keeping in mind that in some countries, travelers might face restrictions on bringing in opioid drugs, even for personal use. A patient on chronic opioids might consider bringing naloxone for the emergency reversal of opioid overdose. Additionally, diabetics should carry glucagon and glucose gel for hypoglycemia management.

In addition to items typically included in a general travel health kit, adventure travelers should consider packing safety equipment to help in an emergency.[1]

Section 19.2 | Travel to High-Risk Areas

TRAVEL ADVISORIES AND SAFETY TIPS

The Department of State (DOS) Bureau of Consular Affairs (BCA) strongly advises against travel to high-risk (Level 4 travel advisory) countries or areas due to dangerous local conditions and the limited ability to assist travelers. Visiting these places can put you at extreme risk.

LOCAL LAWS AND LIMITATIONS ON CONSULAR ASSISTANCE

Be aware that you are subject to the local laws of the countries you visit. Violating these laws can lead to arrest and prosecution, even if the actions are not illegal in the United States. The DOS and BCA often have limited or no capacity to provide assistance in many high-risk areas, particularly during emergencies. Some countries lack a U.S. diplomatic or consular presence, eliminating the possibility of consular services. In select cases, the U.S. cooperates with an official protecting power to offer very limited assistance to U.S. citizens.

WHAT THE STATE DEPARTMENT CAN AND CANNOT DO IN A CRISIS

For details on what assistance can be provided during crises, refer to the State Department's crisis services web page (https://travel.

---

[1] "Adventure Travel," Centers for Disease Control and Prevention (CDC), May 1, 2023. Available online. URL: wwwnc.cdc.gov/travel/yellowbook/2024/work-and-other-reasons/adventure-travel. Accessed July 27, 2024.

state.gov/content/travel/en/international-travel/emergencies/
what-state-dept-can-cant-do-crisis.html).

PRETRAVEL RECOMMENDATIONS
Before traveling to a high-risk area, consider the following steps:

- **Enrollment in travel programs**. Register with the State Department's Smart Traveler Enrollment Program (STEP; https://step.state.gov/step).
- **Communication plans**. Establish a communication plan with your loved ones. Ensure you have a working phone or smart device in your destination to share your location and stay connected.
- **Document sharing**. Share crucial documents, logins, and contacts with someone you trust; they might need this information if your return to the United States is delayed.
- **Contingency planning**. Discuss with loved ones the care and custody of children and property in your absence. Draft a will and designate insurance beneficiaries and power of attorney.
- **Security planning**. Create a personal security plan with your employer or host organization. Consider consulting a professional security firm.
- **Emergency contacts**. Identify essential contacts who can assist in emergencies, such as the nearest U.S. Embassy or Consulate (www.usembassy.gov), the FBI (www.fbi.gov/contact-us/international-offices), and the State Department's Office of American Citizen Services (ACS).
- **Family communication**. Appoint a family member as your contact in case of detention or hostage situations, and establish a proof-of-life protocol.
- **Privacy precautions**. If needed, leave DNA samples with your medical provider for family access, and cleanse your digital presence of sensitive materials that could be perceived as controversial.

PERSONAL SECURITY MEASURES

- **Avoid traveling with valuables.** Leave behind expensive or sentimental items that might be lost or stolen.[1]

Section 19.3 | Travel to Cold Climates

COLD WEATHER RISKS AND PREVENTATIVE MEASURES

You do not have to travel to the Arctic or high altitudes to feel the effects of cold temperatures. Learning how to prevent cold weather injuries and handle potentially dangerous situations caused by the cold is crucial for safety.

PREVENTION OF COLD WEATHER INJURIES

Most cold injuries result from accidents, unexpected severe weather, or inadequate planning. Here are steps to mitigate the risks:

- **Layer your clothing.** Wear warm attire in several loose layers.
- **Choose appropriate outerwear.** Opt for a tightly woven, wind-resistant coat or jacket, and complement it with light, warm inner layers, mittens, hats, and scarves.
- **Select the proper gear.** Ensure your equipment suits the weather, climate, and activities you will undertake.
- **Opt for waterproof footwear.** In wet conditions, wear shoes that are waterproof and offer good traction.
- **Use a suitable wet suit.** For water activities, a thick wet suit is essential to prevent hypothermia.
- **Wear personal flotation devices.** These are vital in aiding those who cannot swim due to injury or cold.
- **Stay dry.** Wet conditions can accelerate heat loss. If active, adjust layers to avoid overheating or sweating excessively.

---

[1] Bureau of Consular Affairs, "High-Risk Area Travelers," U.S. Department of State (DOS), February 26, 2024. Available online. URL: https://travel.state.gov/content/travel/en/international-travel/before-you-go/travelers-with-special-considerations/high-risk-travelers.html. Accessed July 27, 2024.

- **Do not ignore shivering**. Shivering is a preliminary indication of heat loss, and persistent shivering requires finding shelter to warm up.

COMMON COLD INJURIES

Exposure to cold temperatures can rapidly escalate heat loss, leading to conditions such as hypothermia and frostbite, each posing serious health risks.

Hypothermia

Hypothermia occurs when the core body temperature drops below 95 °F (35 °C). While it typically happens in very cold environments, even milder conditions can induce hypothermia if one is wet from rain, sweat, or submersion in cold water.

EARLY SYMPTOMS

- shivering
- fatigue
- clumsiness
- confusion

ADVANCED SYMPTOMS

- cessation of shivering
- blue skin
- dilated pupils
- slowed pulse and breathing
- potential unconsciousness

IMMEDIATE ACTIONS FOR HYPOTHERMIA

- **Seek shelter**. Find a warm indoor area.
- **Remove wet clothing**. Wet clothing contributes to loss of body heat.
- **Warm the core first**. Focus on the chest, neck, head, and groin using warm compresses, or skin-to-skin contact beneath dry layers.

- **Consume warm beverages**. This helps raise the body temperature. Avoid giving beverages to anyone unconscious.

Frostbite

Frostbite occurs from skin exposure to freezing temperatures. It commonly affects the nose, ears, cheeks, chin, fingers, and toes and can cause deep tissue damage.

EARLY SYMPTOMS
- numbness
- tingling
- stinging
- pain

IMMEDIATE ACTIONS FOR HYPOTHERMIA
- Move to a warmer location.
- Remove wet clothing.
- Gently warm or soak the affected area.[1]

Section 19.4 | Travel to Hot Climates

Your chances of getting heat stroke, heat exhaustion, or other heat-related illnesses during travel depend on your destination, activities, level of hydration, and age. Travelers who relax on a beach or by a pool are unlikely to get heat-related illnesses. The more active you are in high temperatures, the more likely you will get a heat-related illness. Learn how to prevent, recognize, and treat heat-related illnesses.

---

[1] "Cold Weather and Travel," Centers for Disease Control and Prevention (CDC), December 12, 2022. Available online. URL: wwwnc.cdc.gov/travel/page/travel-to-cold-climates. Accessed July 27, 2024.

TIPS TO STAY SAFE IN THE HEAT

- **Stay hydrated**. Drink plenty of nonalcoholic fluids.
- **Use sunscreen**. Wear sunscreen with a sun protection factor 15 (SPF 15 or higher) and reapply every two hours or follow the instructions on the package.
- **Wear protective accessories**. Wear a hat and sunglasses.
- **Choose appropriate clothing**. Wear loose, lightweight, light-colored clothing.
- **Plan activities wisely**. Plan outdoor activities during cooler parts of the day.
- **Take breaks**. Rest often and try to stay in the shade when outdoors.
- **Acclimate to the heat**. If you will be doing strenuous activities such as hiking or biking, try to adjust before you travel by exercising one hour per day in the heat.

VULNERABLE GROUPS

The elderly, young children, and people with chronic conditions are more likely to get heat-related illnesses and become ill more quickly compared to healthy adults. However, even young and healthy people can get heat-related illnesses from spending too much time in the heat.

SERIOUS HEAT ILLNESSES

Many heat-related illnesses, such as heat cramps and heat rash, can be treated by getting out of the heat and staying hydrated. However, some can be more serious. It is important to know how to identify signs of serious heat-related illnesses early and get treatment.

HEAT EXHAUSTION

Heat exhaustion is a mild heat-related illness that occurs in hot temperatures and when people do not drink enough water or other nonalcoholic fluids. The elderly, those with high blood pressure, and those working or exercising in the heat are at the highest risk for heat exhaustion.

Symptoms of heat exhaustion include:
- feeling very thirsty
- sweating excessively
- experiencing a headache
- feeling dizzy or confused
- feeling nauseous

If you or anyone you are traveling with has these symptoms, get out of the sun immediately and try to cool off with a fan, air conditioning, or cool water. Also, drink cool, nonalcoholic beverages such as water or sports drinks with electrolytes.

HEAT STROKE

Heat exhaustion can lead to heat stroke, a serious heat-related illness. Heat stroke occurs when the body's temperature rises quickly, and your body cannot cool itself down.

Symptoms of heat stroke include:
- lack of sweating
- high body temperature (rising to 41.11 °C (106 °F) or higher within 10–15 minutes)
- loss of consciousness

Seek medical help immediately. Heat stroke is a medical emergency. It can cause death or permanent disability if emergency treatment is not provided.[1]

[1] "Heat Illnesses," Centers for Disease Control and Prevention (CDC), October 6, 2022. Available online. URL: wwwnc.cdc.gov/travel/page/heat-illnesses. Accessed July 27, 2024.

Chapter 20 | Last-Minute Travel: Ensuring Safety and Health

PRETRAVEL CHECKLIST

Even if you are leaving soon, there are steps you can take to prepare for a safe and healthy trip:

- **Consult the Centers for Disease Control and Prevention (CDC).** The CDC destination pages (wwwnc. cdc.gov/travel/destinations/list) provide important travel health information about your destination, including recommended vaccines and medicines.
- **Schedule a health-care appointment.** If possible, get an in-person or telehealth appointment with your health-care provider to discuss your trip and any vaccinations and medications you may need.
- **Consider accelerated vaccination schedules.** Check with your health-care provider to see if any of the vaccinations you need can be given on an accelerated schedule.
- **Enroll in Smart Traveler Enrollment Program (STEP).** To notify the U.S. Embassy or Consulate of your trip and for help in case of an emergency, enroll in the STEP (https://step.state.gov).

TALK TO YOUR DOCTOR ABOUT VACCINES AND MEDICINES

If you are short on time, some vaccines can be administered on an accelerated schedule, meaning doses are given in a shorter period of time. You may also want to get at least the first dose of certain vaccines that usually require multiple doses to obtain some protection

117

before your trip. These include hepatitis A, Japanese encephalitis, and rabies vaccines.

Yellow Fever Vaccination

Some countries require proof of yellow fever vaccination before entering the country. This proof is usually a signed and stamped International Certificate of Vaccination or Prophylaxis (ICVP) card that you receive after you get the vaccine. Your proof of vaccination is not valid until 10 days after you get it because of the time it takes for your body to build protection. If your destination requires proof of yellow fever vaccination, and you cannot get the vaccine 10 days before travel, you may need to change your travel plans.

Malaria Prevention

If there is a risk of malaria at your destination, your health-care provider may prescribe medicine to prevent malaria. Be sure to let your health-care provider know when you leave, so they can prescribe the right amount of medicine for you. Some malaria medications must be started one to two weeks before you go, while others need to be started only one to two days before you travel. You will still need to take steps to prevent mosquito bites during travel since malaria drugs are not 100 percent effective and do not protect against other diseases spread by mosquitoes such as Zika, dengue, and chikungunya.[1]

SPECIAL CHALLENGES AND ADDITIONAL CONSIDERATIONS
Travelers Leaving in Less than 48 hours

If travel is imminent, clinicians can still provide telehealth or secure digital messaging for prevention counseling and recommendations for services at the destination. During the consultation, emphasize and reassure the last-minute travelers (LMTs) that many travel health risks can be prevented by adhering to healthy behaviors.

---

[1] "Last-Minute Travelers," Centers for Disease Control and Prevention (CDC), August 11, 2022. Available online. URL: wwwnc.cdc.gov/travel/page/last-minute-travelers. Accessed July 26, 2024.

Travelers with Preexisting Medical Conditions

Last-minute travelers with preexisting conditions might be at increased risk for acute episodes of comorbid conditions. These travelers should carry a portable medical record, know reliable sources for medical care at their destination, and purchase travel health insurance, trip insurance, and medical evacuation insurance. Additionally, encourage these travelers to schedule a pretravel appointment or conversation with their treating clinician. Some conditions (such as immunosuppression and pregnancy) often require additional discussion or advanced planning and could warrant delaying departure.

Extended-Stay Travelers

A last-minute consultation will not provide adequate time for a full medical and psychological evaluation or additional education for an expatriate. Advise extended-stay travelers to arrange an early consultation with a qualified clinician at their destination.

Traveler Requests—Carrying Vaccines or Off-Label Dosing

Because of time constraints, some LMTs might ask to carry a vaccine abroad or for a vaccine to be administered off-label (such as a different schedule or double dosing). Due to cold chain concerns, it is rarely advisable to provide travelers with a supplied vaccine. Clinicians who administer a vaccine in a nonstandard manner can face medical-legal issues and induce a false sense of protection in the traveler.

Recurring Last-Minute Travelers

Clinics that frequently see LMTs might want to address this as an administrative issue. The clinical practice could build flexibility into the schedule and proactively identify groups likely to travel last minute (such as college students, corporate employees, and relief workers). For these travelers, the clinic might consider routine pretravel visits or preemptive vaccinations for certain itineraries.[2]

---

[2] "Last-Minute Travelers," Centers for Disease Control and Prevention (CDC), May 1, 2023. Available online. URL: wwwnc.cdc.gov/travel/yellowbook/2024/preparing/last-minute-travelers. Accessed July 26, 2024.

119

TRAVEL TIPS

- **Maintain hand hygiene**. Wash your hands often with soap and clean water, or use hand sanitizer (made with at least 60% alcohol) if clean water is unavailable.
- **Choose safer food and drink options**. Contaminated food or drinks can make you sick with travelers' diarrhea (TD) and other diseases.
- **Use insect repellent**. Wear U.S. Environmental Protection Agency (EPA)-registered insect repellent to prevent mosquito and other bug bites.
- **Dress appropriately**. Consider whether your destination requires preparation for extremely hot or cold weather. For cold weather, bring multiple loose layers and a warm jacket, or light-colored clothing and sunglasses.
- **Avoid animals**. In addition to the risk of rabies, animals can spread other diseases to people.
- **Pack a travel health kit**. Include your prescription and over-the-counter (OTC) medicines. Bring enough medicine to last your whole trip, plus a little extra in case of delays. Also, pack sunscreen with a sun protection factor 15 (SPF 15 or higher) and EPA-registered insect repellent and other supplies.[3]

---

[3] See footnote [1].

Part 3 | **Health Risks during Travel**

Chapter 21 |
Bacterial Infections

Chapter Contents

Section 21.1 | **Brucellosis**

BRUCELLA SPP.: CAUSATIVE AGENTS OF BRUCELLOSIS

Brucella spp. are facultative, intracellular, gram-negative coccobacilli. The primary *Brucella* spp. known to cause human disease include *Brucella abortus* (including the livestock vaccine strain *Brucella abortus* RB51), *Brucella melitensis*, *Brucella suis*, and *Brucella canis*.

EPIDEMIOLOGY AND TRANSMISSION

Over 500,000 new human cases of brucellosis—a bacterial zoonosis—are reported worldwide each year. This figure likely underestimates the actual number due to underreporting and frequent misdiagnoses, as clinical symptoms are nonspecific, physicians may lack awareness, and laboratory capacity for diagnosis is limited. *B. melitensis* is the most frequently reported cause of brucellosis worldwide, but *B. abortus* remains the most widespread potential source of infection.

Human infections most commonly occur among travelers to, or residents of, areas where the disease is endemic in animals—primarily cattle, goats, and sheep—in Africa, Central and South America, Asia, Eastern Europe, the Mediterranean Basin, and the Middle East. In North America, *Brucella* spp. are endemic to the feral swine population and wildlife around the Greater Yellowstone Area.

Humans most commonly acquire *Brucella* by consuming unpasteurized dairy products such as raw milk, butter, soft cheese, or ice cream made from raw milk. The bacteria can also enter the body through skin wounds, mucous membranes, or inhalation, so direct contact with infected animal tissues or fluids poses an exposure risk. Activities such as carcass dressing and assisting birthing animals can increase the risk of contact with infective tissues and fluids.

Travelers' brucellosis can result from *B. suis* or *B. canis* infections, as travelers may contact animal populations infected with these *Brucella* species (e.g., *B. suis* in feral swine and caribou or reindeer, and *B. canis* in dogs). Consumption of undercooked meat from infected animals can lead to infection, though this exposure risk is less likely because bacterial loads are lower in muscle.

Person-to-person transmission has been reported but is rare. Exposure to *Brucella* during pregnancy can increase the risk of miscarriage, so travelers who are or may be pregnant should take extra precautions.

CLINICAL PRESENTATION

The incubation period for brucellosis usually spans two to four weeks, ranging from five days to six months. Initial clinical presentations are nonspecific and include arthralgia, fatigue, fever, headache, malaise, myalgia, and night sweats. Focal infections are common and can affect most organs in the body. Osteoarticular involvement is the most common complication of brucellosis, as is the involvement of the reproductive system. Although rare, endocarditis can occur and is the principal cause of death among patients with brucellosis.

DIAGNOSIS OF BRUCELLOSIS

Blood culture is considered the diagnostic gold standard, but isolation rates can vary considerably (25–80%) depending on the stage of infection, previous use of antimicrobial drugs, type and volume of clinical specimen, and culture method used. Bacterial growth in culture can be observed within three to five days but may take longer; therefore, laboratories should hold cultures for at least 10 days before considering a sample negative.

To increase recovery of the organism, collect samples during a febrile episode and before starting antimicrobial drugs; when focal disease is suspected, collect samples for culture from the affected area (e.g., cerebrospinal fluid (CSF), joint aspirate). Inform the laboratory that brucellosis is suspected when submitting blood, bone marrow, or other clinical specimens for culture because the bacteria take longer to grow, and laboratory personnel require additional personal protective equipment when handling the clinical specimens and culture.

Serologic testing is the most common method for diagnosis. The serum agglutination test (SAT) is the standard method for serologic diagnosis and detects immunoglobulin M (IgM), immunoglobulin G (IgG), and immunoglobulin A (IgA). The Bacterial Special Pathogens Branch at the Centers for Disease Control and Prevention (CDC) performs a modified version of the SAT, known as the "*Brucella* microagglutination test" (BMAT). In general, enzyme-linked immunosorbent assay (ELISA) tests have good sensitivity and specificity and can detect IgM or IgG, and U.S. commercial diagnostic laboratories have the capacity to perform these assays.

Because most *Brucella* serologic assays show variable levels of cross-reactivity with other gram-negative bacteria (e.g., *Escherichia coli* (*E. Coli*) O:157, *Francisella tularensis, Yersinia enterocolitica*), consider the limitations of serologic testing for diagnosing brucellosis. In addition, *Brucella* antibodies can persist for over a year despite successful antibiotic treatment. No validated serologic assays are available to detect antibodies produced against infections caused by *B. canis* and *B. abortus* RB51 strain in humans. If infection with either of these organisms is possible or suspected, perform a culture on a specimen taken before the start of antimicrobial drug therapy.

TREATMENT OF BRUCELLOSIS
A combined regimen of doxycycline (or oral tetracycline) and rifampin for at least six weeks is recommended to treat uncomplicated infection. For complicated brucellosis (endocarditis, meningitis, osteomyelitis), consider adding an aminoglycoside in combination with doxycycline and extend the duration of therapy to four to six months. *B. abortus* RB51 is resistant to rifampin; modify treatment for brucellosis caused by this strain accordingly (e.g., doxycycline in combination with trimethoprim-sulfamethoxazole, unless contraindicated). Other antimicrobial agents have been used in various combinations; a clinician with expertise in infectious diseases should guide treatment. Incorrect or incomplete therapy or late diagnosis can result in relapse.

PREVENTION OF BRUCELLOSIS
Travelers should avoid unpasteurized dairy products, undercooked meat, and potentially contaminated meat products in countries where

brucellosis is endemic. People who dress or butcher wild animals or who handle birthing products from animals potentially infected with *Brucella* spp. should wear appropriate protective equipment, including rubber gloves, goggles or face shields, and gowns. Inform clinical microbiology laboratories when submitting specimens from patients with suspected brucellosis to ensure proper biosafety precautions in handling specimens and specimen derivatives.[1]

Section 21.2 | Cholera

Cholera is an acute bacterial intestinal infection caused by toxigenic *Vibrio cholerae* O-group 1 (O1) or O-group 139 (O139). Many other serogroups of *V. cholerae*, with or without the cholera toxin gene (including the nontoxigenic strains of the O1 and O139 serogroups), can cause a cholera-like illness. Only toxigenic strains of serogroups O1 and O139 have caused widespread epidemics and are reportable to the World Health Organization (WHO) as "cholera." Toxigenic strains of *V. cholerae* O1 are the source of an ongoing global pandemic that began in 1961, but the O139 serogroup is localized to a few areas in Asia.

Vibrio cholerae O1 has two biotypes, classical and El Tor, and each biotype can be divided into distinct serotypes, Inaba, Ogawa, and, rarely, Hikojima. The symptoms of infection are indistinguishable, but more people infected with the El Tor biotype remain asymptomatic or have only a mild illness. Globally, most cholera cases are caused by O1 El Tor organisms. An El Tor variant with characteristics of both classical and El Tor biotypes has emerged in Asia and spread to Africa and the Caribbean. This strain is responsible for the epidemic on Hispaniola, the island shared by Haiti and the Dominican Republic; compared to older El Tor strains, this newer variant appears to be more virulent, causing a greater

---

[1] "Brucellosis," Centers for Disease Control and Prevention (CDC), May 1, 2023. Available online. URL: wwwnc. cdc.gov/travel/yellowbook/2024/infections-diseases/brucellosis. Accessed April 3, 2024.

proportion of severe episodes of cholera with the potential for higher death rates.

TRANSMISSION OF CHOLERA

Toxigenic *V. cholerae* O1 and O139 are free-living bacterial organisms found in fresh and brackish water, often associated with copepods or other zooplankton, shellfish, and aquatic plants. Cholera infections are most often acquired from untreated drinking water in which toxigenic *V. cholerae* naturally occurs or has been introduced from the feces of an infected person. Other common vehicles include raw or undercooked seafood, especially fish and shellfish. Other foods, including produce, are less commonly implicated. Direct person-to-person transmission, including to health-care workers during epidemics, has been reported.

When in countries affected by cholera, travelers who consistently observe recommendations regarding safe drinking water, food preparation and consumption, handwashing, and sanitation have virtually no risk of acquiring the disease.

EPIDEMIOLOGY OF CHOLERA

Cholera is endemic to approximately 50 countries, primarily in South and Southeast Asia and Africa. During 2007–2017, the United States had 117 confirmed cholera cases among people who traveled internationally in the week before illness; approximately 16 percent reported travel to India or Pakistan. Other reported destinations included other countries in Southeast Asia, East and West Africa, and the Caribbean. Sporadic cases in the United States associated with travel to or from cholera-affected countries in Asia and Africa continue to occur.

Approximately, 60 percent of U.S. cases during 2007–2017 were linked to travel to Haiti, the Dominican Republic, or Cuba, the three Caribbean countries affected by a large cholera epidemic that began in Haiti in October 2010. Ninety-four percent of case-patients reported travel to either Haiti or the Dominican Republic sometime during 2010–2017. The other case-patients had been to Cuba sometime during 2013–2015.

In 2018 and 2019, the most recent years for which data are available, no cholera cases in the United States were associated with travel to Haiti or the Dominican Republic, and those two countries reported far fewer cholera cases to WHO during these two years than in previous years. Although efforts were underway to eliminate cholera from Hispaniola, in October 2022, the Pan American Health Organization (PAHO) reported a resurgence of the disease in Haiti. Before 2022, the last confirmed case of cholera in Haiti was in 2019, and in the Dominican Republic in 2018.

Travelers to areas where cholera is endemic or where an active epidemic is occurring are at risk for cholera infection. Health care and response workers in cholera-affected areas (e.g., during an outbreak or after a disaster) also might be at increased risk for cholera. People who do not follow handwashing recommendations, and/or do not use latrines or other sanitation systems are at increased risk for infection. People who have low gastric acidity have a greater risk for infection, and they, along with those with blood type O, are at greater risk for developing severe disease if infected.

CLINICAL PRESENTATION

Cholera most commonly manifests as acute watery diarrhea in an afebrile person. The pathogen typically remains in the gastrointestinal (GI) tract and does not invade the bloodstream. Infection is often mild or asymptomatic, but it can be severe. Severe cholera (cholera gravis) occurs in approximately 10 percent of cholera episodes and is characterized by profuse watery diarrhea, described as rice-water stools, often accompanied by nausea and vomiting that can rapidly lead to severe volume depletion.

Clinical findings include dry mucous membranes and loss of skin turgor, hypotension, tachycardia, and thirst. Additional symptoms, including muscle cramps, are secondary to the resulting electrolyte imbalances. Untreated cholera can cause rapid loss of body fluids, which can lead to severe dehydration, hypovolemic shock, and death within hours. The case-fatality ratio for untreated cholera can reach more than 50 percent, but with adequate and timely rehydration, the case-fatality ratio is less than 1 percent.

DIAGNOSIS OF CHOLERA

In the United States, cholera traditionally is confirmed by isolation and identification of toxigenic *V. cholerae* O1 recovered from a stool sample of a patient with acute, watery diarrhea. Before administering antimicrobial treatment, collect patient stool samples and preserve samples in Cary-Blair medium for transport at ambient temperature. Selective media (e.g., taurocholate-tellurite-gelatin agar, thiosulfate-citrate-bile salts agar) also can be used for pathogen isolation.

Cholera is a nationally notifiable disease in the United States, and all isolates obtained in the United States should be sent to the Centers for Disease Control and Prevention (CDC) via state health department laboratories for identification and virulence testing.

TREATMENT OF CHOLERA

Rehydration is the cornerstone of cholera treatment. Administer oral rehydration solution and, when necessary, intravenous fluids and electrolytes; timely administration in adequate volumes will reduce case-fatality ratios to less than 1 percent. Antibiotics will reduce fluid requirements and duration of illness and are indicated in conjunction with aggressive hydration for severe cases and for patients with moderate dehydration and ongoing fluid losses.

Antimicrobial susceptibility testing should inform treatment choices whenever possible. In most countries, doxycycline is recommended as the first-line antibiotic treatment for children, adults, and pregnant people. Previously, tetracycline antibiotics (including doxycycline) were not recommended for children due to concern for dental discoloration or pregnant people due to concern for teratogenic effects. A systematic review among young children and pregnant people receiving doxycycline did not demonstrate a safety risk.

Multidrug-resistant isolates are emerging, particularly in South Asia, with resistance to quinolones, trimethoprim-sulfamethoxazole, and tetracycline. The strain from Hispaniola is also multidrug resistant; as of 2013, however, tested isolates were still sensitive to doxycycline and tetracycline. Macrolides, including erythromycin and azithromycin, are alternative agents for multidrug-resistant isolates. Zinc supplementation reduces the severity and duration of cholera and other diarrheal diseases in children living in resource-limited areas.

PREVENTION OF CHOLERA
Food and Water
Travelers should follow safe food and water precautions and frequently wash their hands. Antibiotic chemoprophylaxis is not recommended.

Vaccine
No country or territory requires vaccination against cholera as a condition for entry. CVD 103-HgR, a live, attenuated, single-dose oral cholera vaccine (Vaxchora*, PaxVax), is licensed in the United States. The vaccine was previously marketed under the names Orochol and Mutacol in other countries.

Vaxchora is not currently licensed for use in children <2 years or adults >65 years of age.

Cholera continues to pose a global health challenge, particularly in regions lacking proper sanitation. Effective management, including surveillance, vaccination, and public education, is vital for controlling outbreaks and reducing transmission. A multifaceted approach integrating medical and infrastructural improvements is crucial for eradicating this preventable disease.[1]

Section 21.3 | Leptospirosis

LEPTOSPIRA SPP.: THE CAUSATIVE AGENT OF LEPTOSPIROSIS
Leptospira spp. are obligate aerobic, gram-negative spirochete bacteria responsible for leptospirosis.

TRANSMISSION OF LEPTOSPIROSIS
Leptospira transmit through abrasions or cuts in the skin, the conjunctiva, and mucous membranes. Macerated skin, resulting from prolonged water exposure, is another suspected route

---

[1] "Cholera," Centers for Disease Control and Prevention (CDC), May 1, 2023. Available online. URL: wwwnc.cdc.gov/travel/yellowbook/2024/infections-diseases/cholera. Accessed April 3, 2024.

of infection. Humans can be infected by direct contact with urine or reproductive fluids from infected animals, contact with urine-contaminated freshwater sources or wet soil, or by consuming contaminated food or water. Infection rarely occurs through animal bites or human-to-human contact. Rodents are an important reservoir for *Leptospira*, but most mammals, including dogs, horses, cattle, swine, and many wildlife species, can be infected and shed the bacteria in their urine.

EPIDEMIOLOGY OF LEPTOSPIROSIS

Leptospirosis is distributed worldwide; however, its incidence is greater in tropical climates. Regions with the highest estimated morbidity and mortality include parts of sub-Saharan Africa, Latin America, the Caribbean, South and Southeast Asia, and Oceania. Travelers to endemic areas are at increased risk when participating in recreational freshwater activities, such as boating and swimming, particularly after heavy rainfall or flooding. Prolonged exposure to contaminated water and activities that involve head immersion or swallowing water increase the risk for infection.

Participating in activities involving mud, such as adventure races, also increases a traveler's risk for infection, as does working directly with animals in endemic areas, especially when exposed to their body fluids, and visiting or residing in areas with rodent infestation. Leptospirosis occurs most commonly in adult males. The estimated worldwide annual incidence exceeds 1 million cases, including approximately 59,000 deaths.

Outbreaks can occur after heavy rainfall or flooding in endemic areas, especially in urban areas of low- and middle-income countries, where housing conditions and sanitation are poor and rodent infestation is common. Outbreaks of leptospirosis have occurred after flooding in popular U.S. travel destinations, including Florida, Hawaii, Puerto Rico, and the U.S. Virgin Islands. Nearly half of the leptospirosis cases reported in the continental United States during 2014–2018, with an identified geographic source of infection, were associated with international travel. Most U.S. cases are reported outside the continental United States in the domestic travel destinations of Hawaii and Puerto Rico.

CLINICAL PRESENTATION

The incubation period for leptospirosis ranges from 2 to 30 days, but illness usually occurs 5–14 days after exposure. Most infections are asymptomatic, but clinical illness can present as a self-limiting acute febrile illness, estimated to occur in approximately 90 percent of clinical infections, or as a severe, potentially fatal illness with multiorgan dysfunction in 5–10 percent of patients. In patients who progress to severe disease, the illness can be biphasic, with a temporary decrease in fever between phases.

The acute, septicemic phase lasts about seven days and presents as an acute febrile illness with symptoms including severe headache, photophobia, retro-orbital pain, chills, myalgias (particularly in the calves and lower back), conjunctival suffusion (characteristic of leptospirosis but not occurring in all cases), nausea, vomiting, diarrhea, abdominal pain, cough, and, rarely, a skin rash.

The second or immune phase is characterized by antibody production and the presence of leptospires in the urine. In patients who progress to severe disease, clinical findings can include cardiac arrhythmias, hemodynamic collapse, hemorrhage, jaundice, liver failure, aseptic meningitis, pulmonary insufficiency, and renal failure. The classically described syndrome, Weil disease, consists of renal and liver failure.

Among patients with severe disease, the case-fatality ratio ranges from 5 to 15 percent. Severe pulmonary hemorrhagic syndrome is a rare but severe form of leptospirosis that can have a case-fatality ratio exceeding 50 percent. Poor prognostic indicators include older age, development of altered mental status, respiratory insufficiency, or oliguria.

DIAGNOSIS OF LEPTOSPIROSIS

Submit a combination of samples for leptospirosis testing, including serum samples; whenever possible, obtain acute and convalescent sample pairs. During early disease, polymerase chain reaction (PCR) analysis of whole blood (collected in the first week of illness) and urine (collected after the first week of illness) can be helpful. PCR analysis of cerebrospinal fluid (CSF) also can be helpful in diagnosing patients with signs of meningitis.

Diagnosis of leptospirosis is often based on serology; the microscopic agglutination test (MAT) is the reference standard and can only be performed at certain reference laboratories. Various serologic screening tests are available at commercial laboratories, including enzyme-linked immunosorbent assay (ELISA) and ImmunoDOT/DotBlot rapid diagnostic tests. The use of immunoglobulin M (IgM)-specific serologic screening tests is recommended, and positive screening tests should be confirmed with MAT.

Detection of the organism in acute whole blood using real-time PCR can provide a more timely diagnosis during the early, septicemic phase, and PCR also can be performed on CSF or convalescent urine. A positive PCR result is confirmatory for infection. Culture is insensitive, slow, and requires special media; it is therefore not recommended as the sole diagnostic method.

The Zoonoses and Select Agent Laboratory (ZSAL) at the Centers for Disease Control and Prevention (CDC) performs MAT and PCR for diagnosis of leptospirosis as well as culture identification and genotyping of isolates.

TREATMENT OF LEPTOSPIROSIS
If leptospirosis is suspected, initiate antimicrobial therapy as soon as possible, without waiting for diagnostic test results. Early treatment can be effective in decreasing the severity and duration of infection. For patients with mild symptoms, doxycycline is the drug of choice, unless contraindicated; alternative options include ampicillin, amoxicillin, or azithromycin. Intravenous penicillin is the drug of choice for patients with severe leptospirosis; ceftriaxone and cefotaxime are alternative antimicrobial agents.

PREVENTION OF LEPTOSPIROSIS
The best way to prevent infection is to avoid exposure. Advise travelers to avoid exposure to potentially contaminated bodies of freshwater, floodwaters, potentially infected animals or their body fluids, and areas with rodent infestation. Educate travelers who might be at increased risk for infection to consider taking additional preventive

measures, such as wearing protective clothing, especially footwear, instructing them to cover cuts and abrasions with occlusive dressings, counseling them on boiling or chemically treating potentially contaminated drinking water, and providing chemoprophylaxis. No human vaccine is available in the United States.[1]

Section 21.4 | Tetanus

CLOSTRIDIUM TETANI: CAUSATIVE AGENT OF TETANUS

Clostridium tetani, a spore-forming, anaerobic, gram-positive bacterium, is the causative agent of tetanus. Ubiquitous in the environment, spores of *C. tetani* germinate into toxin-producing bacteria under specific conditions when they enter the body.

TRANSMISSION OF TETANUS

Tetanus is transmitted via direct contamination of open wounds and non-intact skin. Non-neonatal tetanus is typically acquired when spores enter wounds contaminated with dirt, animal or human excreta or saliva, or necrotic tissue. Burns, crush injuries, and deep punctures are also at increased risk for tetanus infection. Even wounds without visible contamination can become infected with tetanus spores; transmission has been associated with abortion, dental infection, injection drug use, otitis media, pregnancy, and surgery. Neonatal tetanus is typically acquired when spores contaminate the umbilical cord due to unhygienic delivery practices. Direct person-to-person transmission does not occur.

EPIDEMIOLOGY OF TETANUS

Tetanus is distributed worldwide. It is more prevalent in rural and agricultural regions, areas where contact with soil or animal excreta is likely, warm and moist environments, and areas

---

[1] "Leptospirosis," Centers for Disease Control and Prevention (CDC), May 1, 2023. Available online. URL: wwwnc. cdc.gov/travel/yellowbook/2024/infections-diseases/leptospirosis. Accessed July 27, 2024.

where immunization against tetanus is inadequate. Because the spores exist in the environment, tetanus cannot be eradicated. In 2020, over 11,750 tetanus cases globally were reported to the World Health Organization (WHO)/United Nations Children's Fund (UNICEF), including 2,230 neonatal cases. Most cases were reported from countries in Africa and Southeast Asia.

Maternal and neonatal tetanus elimination, defined as fewer than one neonatal tetanus case per 1,000 live births per year in every district of a country, has not been achieved in Afghanistan, Angola, Central African Republic, Guinea, Mali, Nigeria, Pakistan, Papua New Guinea, Somalia, Sudan, South Sudan, or Yemen. Travelers not up-to-date with tetanus vaccination are at risk of acquiring tetanus infection. Hygienic obstetric care might not be available in countries that have not eliminated maternal and neonatal tetanus, increasing the risk for morbidity and mortality from tetanus infection; in addition, proper wound management and tetanus immune globulin (TIG) are less likely to be available in these settings.

Tetanus can affect any age group. The risk for injuries after natural disasters is high; therefore, humanitarian aid workers should be up-to-date on tetanus vaccination before travel. The number of U.S. travelers who acquire tetanus infection abroad is unknown; surveillance might be limited because travelers with injuries are unlikely to seek care at a travel clinic upon their return. Injuries are common among travelers, however, and any tetanus-prone wound is a risk, so ensure that all travelers are properly vaccinated.

CLINICAL PRESENTATION

The average incubation period for tetanus is 10 days (range 3–21 days). The duration of the incubation period is inversely related to the severity of symptoms, with shorter incubation periods associated with injuries closer to the central nervous system (CNS). Tetanus is classified as generalized, localized, and cephalic. Generalized tetanus, occurring in more than 80 percent of cases, is characterized by lockjaw, generalized spasms, risus sardonicus, and opisthotonus. Symptoms of localized tetanus include muscle spasms confined to the injury site. Cephalic tetanus is characterized by a head or face wound and flaccid cranial nerve palsies.

Progression from localized and cephalic to generalized tetanus can occur. Neonatal tetanus occurs in newborns who have contaminated umbilical stumps and whose mothers are unimmunized or inadequately immunized. Neonatal tetanus can lead to long-term sequelae, including behavioral, intellectual, and neurologic abnormalities. Severe tetanus can lead to respiratory failure and death. Case-fatality ratios for generalized tetanus vary between 25 and 100 percent and can be reduced to 10–20 percent where modern intensive care is available. The case-fatality ratio is less than 1 percent for localized tetanus.

DIAGNOSIS OF TETANUS

Diagnosis is based on clinical findings with epidemiologic support; no confirmatory laboratory tests are available. Tetanus is a nationally notifiable disease in the United States.

TREATMENT OF TETANUS

The treatment goals are to inactivate circulating toxin by immediately administering TIG, eliminate the bacteria with aggressive wound care and debridement to stop further toxin formation, provide supportive care, and provide antibiotic treatment for 7–10 days. Metronidazole is the most appropriate antibiotic; parenteral penicillin G is an alternative treatment. Patients with tetanus must be hospitalized in a quiet, dim room to minimize spasms. Additional supportive care measures include agents to control muscle spasms and autonomic dysfunction, and respiratory support.

PREVENTION OF TETANUS

Vaccination is the only prevention against tetanus. Because immunity after vaccination wanes over time, lifelong vaccination with tetanus toxoid–containing vaccine (TTCV) is necessary to attain and sustain immunity against tetanus. All travelers should be up-to-date with vaccination before departure.

Children should receive diphtheria-tetanus-acellular pertussis (DTaP) and diphtheria-tetanus (DT) for those less than seven years, while tetanus-diphtheria-acellular pertussis (Tdap) and tetanus-diphtheria (Td) are indicated for children aged 10 years and older. Infants and children should receive five doses of DTaP at 2, 4, 6, and 15–18 months, and at 4–6 years; adolescents should receive one dose of Tdap at 11–12 years of age. Children aged 7 years and older can receive Tdap for catch-up vaccination.

Adults should receive TTCV booster doses every 10 years. Adults who have never received Tdap should do so; otherwise, clinicians can administer either Td or Tdap. Previously unvaccinated pregnant people should receive two doses of TTCV during their pregnancy. Pregnant people should also be properly vaccinated to prevent infant pertussis, irrespective of their vaccination history, by receiving Tdap during every pregnancy at 27–36 weeks gestation, preferably earlier in this period.

Adverse reactions to TTCVs are generally mild and include fatigue, headache, and injection site pain. A severe allergic reaction (e.g., anaphylaxis) to a previous dose or a vaccine component is a contraindication for any TTCV. For DTaP or Tdap, encephalopathy without an identifiable cause occurring within seven days of a previous dose is a contraindication. Precautions for all TTCV include Guillain-Barré syndrome (GBS) within 6 weeks after a previous dose, a history of Arthus-type hypersensitivity after a previous dose (in which case, vaccination should be deferred until at least 10 years after the last TTCV), and moderate or severe acute illness with or without fever.[1]

Section 21.5 | Travelers' Diarrhea

WHAT IS TRAVELERS' DIARRHEA?

Travelers' diarrhea (TD) is the most common travel-related illness, particularly prevalent in Asia (excluding Japan and South Korea), the Middle East, Africa, Mexico, and Central and South America.

---

[1] "Tetanus," Centers for Disease Control and Prevention (CDC), May 1, 2023. Available online. URL: wwwnc.cdc. gov/travel/yellowbook/2024/infections-diseases/tetanus. Accessed July 29, 2024.

Although diarrhea is rarely serious or life-threatening in otherwise healthy adults, it can significantly disrupt travel plans.

STEPS TO AVOID TRAVELERS' DIARRHEA

- **Choose food and drinks carefully**. Consume only foods that are cooked and served hot. Avoid food that has been sitting on a buffet. Eat raw fruits and vegetables only if you have washed them in clean water or peeled them yourself. Drink only beverages from factory-sealed containers and avoid ice, as it may have been made from unclean water.
- **Wash your hands**. Frequently wash your hands with soap and water, especially after using the bathroom and before eating. If soap and water are not available, use an alcohol-based hand sanitizer. Generally, avoid putting your hands near your mouth.

WAYS TO TREAT TRAVELERS' DIARRHEA

- **Stay hydrated**. If you develop diarrhea, it is crucial to drink plenty of fluids to prevent dehydration. For severe cases of TD, consider using an oral rehydration solution, which is available online or in pharmacies in developing countries, for fluid replacement.
- **Use over-the-counter (OTC) drugs**. Drugs like loperamide, available OTC, can reduce the frequency and urgency of bowel movements. These medications may facilitate easier travel, such as riding on a bus or airplane, while waiting for antibiotics to take effect.
- **Consider antibiotics judiciously**. Your doctor may prescribe antibiotics for TD; however, reserve these for severe cases. Follow your doctor's instructions precisely when taking antibiotics. If severe diarrhea begins soon after returning from your trip, consult a doctor and request stool tests to determine the most effective antibiotic treatment.

While TD can disrupt travel plans, taking preventive steps and knowing how to treat symptoms can help minimize discomfort and ensure a more enjoyable trip. Always prioritize hygiene and safe eating practices to reduce the risk of TD.[1]

Section 21.6 | Tuberculosis

MYCOBACTERIUM TUBERCULOSIS COMPLEX

Mycobacterium tuberculosis complex is a group of closely related rod-shaped, nonmotile, slow-growing, acid-fast bacteria. It includes *Mycobacterium bovis* and *M. tuberculosis* hominins, the most common cause of human tuberculosis (TB), often referred to as "*M. tuberculosis*."

TRANSMISSION OF TUBERCULOSIS

Transmission occurs when a person with a contagious form of the infection coughs, spreading bacilli through the air. Bovine TB, caused by *M. bovis*, is acquired by consuming unpasteurized dairy products from infected cattle.

The risk for *M. tuberculosis* transmission on an airplane is low, but instances of in-flight TB transmission have occurred. The risk depends on the contagiousness of the infected individual, seating proximity, flight duration, and host factors. To prevent transmission, individuals with contagious TB should not travel by commercial airplanes or other commercial conveyances. Typically, only TB of the lung or airway is contagious in community contexts. Health department authorities determine whether TB is contagious based on a person's chest radiograph, sputum tests, symptoms, and treatment received. The World Health Organization (WHO) has issued guidelines for notifying passengers potentially exposed to TB on airplanes. Passengers concerned about possible TB exposure should

---

[1] "Travelers' Diarrhea," Centers for Disease Control and Prevention (CDC), May 3, 2022. Available online. URL: wwwnc.cdc.gov/travel/page/travelers-diarrhea. Accessed July 29, 2024.

consult their primary health-care provider or visit their local health department clinic for evaluation.

Bovine TB is a risk for travelers who consume unpasteurized dairy products in countries where *M. bovis* in cattle is common, such as Mexico. The risk in some African countries has been postulated, but human *M. bovis* statistics are unavailable for those regions.

EPIDEMIOLOGY OF TUBERCULOSIS

According to the WHO, approximately 10 million new TB cases and about 1.2 million TB-related deaths occurred in 2019. TB is prevalent worldwide, but the incidence varies. In some countries in sub-Saharan Africa and Asia, the annual incidence is several hundred per 100,000 population. In the United States, the annual incidence is less than three per 100,000 population, but immigrants from countries with a high TB burden and long-term residents of high-burden countries have a tenfold greater incidence of TB than the U.S. national average. U.S. surveillance does not capture travel-related cases of TB.

Drug-resistant TB is an increasing concern. Multidrug-resistant (MDR) TB is resistant to at least the two most effective drugs, isoniazid and rifampin. MDR TB is less common than drug-susceptible TB, but globally approximately 363,000 cases of MDR TB were diagnosed in 2019, and MDR TB accounts for more than 25 percent of TB cases in some countries. MDR and higher-order resistance are of particular concern among individuals infected with HIV or other immunocompromised people.

CLINICAL PRESENTATION

Mycobacterium tuberculosis infection can be detected by a positive tuberculin skin test (TST) or interferon-γ release assay (IGRA) 8–10 weeks after exposure. Overall, only 5–10 percent of otherwise healthy people who are infected progress to TB disease during their lifetimes. Progression to TB disease can take weeks to decades after initial infection. People with TB disease have symptoms or other manifestations of illness (e.g., an abnormal chest radiograph). For most people who become infected, *M. tuberculosis* remains inactive (latent TB infection or LTBI), in which the infected person has no symptoms and cannot spread the infection to others.

TB disease can affect any organ but affects the lungs in 70–80 percent of cases. Typical symptoms include prolonged cough, fever, hemoptysis, night sweats, decreased appetite, and weight loss. The most common sites for extrapulmonary TB are the bladder, bones and joints, brain and meninges, genitalia, kidneys, lymph nodes, and pleura.

The risk for progression to disease is much higher in immuno-suppressed people; for example, progression is 8–10 percent per year in HIV-infected people not receiving antiretroviral therapy (ART). People receiving tumor necrosis factor blockers to treat rheumatoid arthritis (RA) and other chronic inflammatory conditions also are at increased risk for disease progression.

DIAGNOSIS OF TUBERCULOSIS
Pre- and Post-Travel Testing
Before leaving the United States, travelers who anticipate possible prolonged exposure to TB should have a pretravel Interferon-Gamma Release Assay (IGRA). This includes people who will care for patients or work in health-care facilities, prisons, jails, refugee camps, or homeless shelters, and those planning prolonged stays in TB-endemic countries. If the predeparture test is negative, repeat the IGRA or single TST 8–10 weeks after returning. The predeparture and follow-up tests should be the same type to facilitate the interpretation of results. People with HIV infection or other immunocompromising conditions are more likely to have an impaired response to either a skin or blood test.

Medical Evaluation
Travelers who suspect they have been exposed to TB should inform their health-care provider of the possible exposure and receive a medical evaluation. Because drug resistance is relatively common in some parts of the world, consult with experts in infectious diseases or pulmonary medicine regarding proper management and coordinate consultations with input from the public health department.

TREATMENT OF TUBERCULOSIS
Latent Tuberculosis Infection
People with LTBI can be treated, and treatments are effective at preventing the progression of TB disease. Clinicians must exclude TB disease before starting LTBI treatment. In the United States, several regimens exist for the treatment of drug-susceptible LTBI. Choose a regimen based on coexisting medical conditions, potential for drug interactions, and drug-susceptibility results of the presumed source of exposure, if known.

Tuberculosis Disease
The CDC, American Thoracic Society (ATS), and Infectious Diseases Society of America (IDSA) have published guidelines for treating drug-susceptible TB disease with a multiple-drug regimen administered by directly observed therapy for six to nine months. Drug-resistant TB is more difficult to treat, historically requiring 4–6 drugs for 18–24 months, and is best managed by an expert.

PREVENTION OF TUBERCULOSIS
Travelers should avoid exposure to people with TB disease in crowded and enclosed environments. Based on WHO recommendations, the Bacillus Calmette-Guérin (BCG) vaccine is used once, at birth, in countries with higher TB burdens to reduce the severe consequences of TB in infants and children. BCG vaccine has low and variable efficacy in preventing TB in adults. All people, including those who have received BCG vaccination, must follow recommended TB infection control precautions to the greatest extent possible. IGRA is preferred over TST for pre- and post-travel testing in those vaccinated with BCG because BCG might induce false-positive TST results.

To prevent infections from *M. bovis* and other foodborne pathogens, travelers should avoid consuming unpasteurized dairy products.[1]

---

[1] "Tuberculosis," Centers for Disease Control and Prevention (CDC), May 1, 2023. Available online. URL: wwwnc.cdc.gov/travel/yellowbook/2024/infections-diseases/tuberculosis. Accessed July 29, 2024.

Section 21.7 | Typhoid and Paratyphoid Fevers

Typhoid and paratyphoid fevers are similar illnesses caused by different bacteria: *Salmonella* Typhi and *Salmonella* Paratyphi, respectively. These diseases are transmitted through contaminated food and water, often in settings where sanitation and hygiene practices are inadequate.

TRANSMISSION OF THE BACTERIA

Individuals infected with these bacteria can spread them, typically through poor hygiene practices. This occurs when an infected person handles food or beverages without washing their hands after using the bathroom. In regions with substandard sanitation, water used for washing and preparing food, including tap water, can also become contaminated, posing a risk to anyone who consumes it.

WHO IS AT RISK?

Typhoid and paratyphoid fevers are prevalent in areas with unsafe water and food supplies, particularly in Eastern and Southern Asia, Africa, the Caribbean, Central and South America, and the Middle East. Travelers visiting friends or relatives in these regions face a higher risk due to potentially prolonged exposure and less cautious consumption of local food and water.

Annually in the United States, around 425 people are diagnosed with typhoid fever and about 125 with paratyphoid fever. Most of these individuals have traveled internationally.

SYMPTOMS OF TYPHOID AND PARATYPHOID FEVERS

Both diseases typically present with high fever, reaching up to 103–104 °F (39–40 °C), and can include weakness, stomach pain, headache, diarrhea or constipation, cough, and loss of appetite. Some individuals may develop a rash of flat, rose-colored spots. While rare, these infections can lead to severe complications, such as internal bleeding and death.

PREVENTION STRATEGIES

The best ways to prevent typhoid and paratyphoid fevers include vaccination, cautious selection of food and drinks, and rigorous hand hygiene.

Vaccination Options

- **Pill vaccine.** This vaccine is suitable for individuals six years and older and requires completion of all four doses at least one week before travel.
- **Injection vaccine.** Available for those two years and older, it should be administered at least two weeks before departure.

Discuss these vaccines with a health-care provider well before traveling, as they are only 50–80 percent effective. Since no vaccine is available for paratyphoid fever, meticulous attention to food and beverage selection remains crucial.

Safe Food and Drink Practices

- Consume only food that is cooked and served hot.
- Avoid buffet-style food that has been left out.
- Only eat fruits and vegetables you have washed in clean water or peeled yourself.
- Drink beverages only from factory-sealed containers and avoid unpasteurized milk.
- Do not consume ice, as it may be made from contaminated water.

Hand Hygiene

- Wash your hands regularly with soap and water for at least 20 seconds, particularly after using the bathroom and before eating.
- If soap and water are unavailable, use an alcohol-based hand sanitizer with at least 60 percent alcohol content.
- Avoid touching your face and mouth to prevent the transfer of bacteria.

Bacterial Infections

By understanding the risks and actively engaging in preventative measures, travelers can significantly reduce their chances of contracting typhoid or paratyphoid fever. Maintaining high standards of personal hygiene and being cautious with food and drink choices are crucial steps in ensuring a safe and healthy travel experience.[1]

[1] "Typhoid Fever," Centers for Disease Control and Prevention (CDC), June 2, 2023. Available online. URL: wwwnc. cdc.gov/travel/diseases/typhoid. Accessed April July 29, 2024.

Chapter 22 |
Viral Infections

Chapter Contents

Section 22.1 | Chikungunya

WHAT IS CHIKUNGUNYA?
Chikungunya is a viral disease transmitted to humans by the bite of infected mosquitoes. The virus circulates between humans and mosquitoes, with mosquitoes becoming infectious after feeding on a person carrying the virus. These mosquitoes can transmit the virus to other individuals through their bites.

WHO IS AT RISK?
Chikungunya virus is spread by mosquitoes found in many regions worldwide, including Africa, Asia, the Americas, and islands in the Indian and Pacific Oceans. These mosquitoes are active and can bite both during the day and at night, putting travelers to these areas at risk of infection.

SYMPTOMS OF CHIKUNGUNYA
Symptoms typically appear three to seven days after an infected mosquito bite and include fever and joint pain. Other symptoms may include headache, muscle pain, joint swelling, and rash. While most people recover within a week, some may experience prolonged joint pain that can last for months.

PREVENTIVE MEASURES FOR TRAVELERS
Travelers can reduce their risk of chikungunya infection by taking several proactive steps:
- **Use EPA-registered insect repellent**. Opt for insect repellents approved by the Environmental Protection Agency (EPA) containing active ingredients such as N,N-diethyl-meta-toluamide (DEET), picaridin, IR3535, oil of lemon eucalyptus (OLE), para-menthane-diol (PMD), or 2-undecanone. These repellents are deemed safe and effective, including for pregnant and breastfeeding women. Always apply repellent after sunscreen.

Find the suitable repellent using the EPA's search tool at www.epa.gov/insect-repellents/find-repellent-right-you.

- **Insect repellent usage for babies and children.**
  - Ensure children wear clothing covering their arms and legs.
  - Use mosquito netting over strollers and baby carriers.
  - Always follow product label instructions and avoid using products with OLE or PMD on children under three years old.
  - Avoid applying repellent to children's hands, eyes, mouth, or irritated skin. Instead, adults should apply repellent to their hands and then to the child's face.
  - Wear protective clothing. Dress in long-sleeved shirts and long pants.
- **Treat clothing and gear with permethrin.** Apply 0.5 percent permethrin to clothing and gear or purchase items already treated. Permethrin acts as an insecticide, providing protection even after multiple washings. Follow the product instructions carefully and avoid applying permethrin directly to the skin.
- **Secure your lodging.** Choose accommodations with air conditioning or screens on windows and doors to keep mosquitoes out. Use a mosquito net if such features are not available or if sleeping outdoors.
- **Sleeping arrangements.** Use a mosquito net, especially when sleeping in areas without protective screens. Ensure the net is compact, white, rectangular, with 156 holes per square inch, and long enough to tuck under the mattress. Permethrin-treated nets offer enhanced protection against mosquitoes.

Travelers can significantly mitigate their risk of contracting chikungunya through vigilant preventive measures, including using

EPA-registered insect repellents, wearing appropriate clothing, and ensuring safe accommodations. Understanding these precautions and implementing them can help travelers enjoy their journeys without the burden of illness.[1]

Section 22.2 | COVID-19

WHAT IS COVID-19

Coronavirus 2019 (COVID-19) is a respiratory illness caused by the severe acute respiratory syndrome coronavirus 2 (SARS-CoV-2). The virus primarily spreads through respiratory droplets and small particles produced when an infected person coughs, sneezes, or talks, particularly in crowded or poorly ventilated indoor settings.

SYMPTOMS OF COVID-19

Symptoms range from none or mild to severe and may appear 2–14 days after exposure to the virus. These can include:
- fever
- chills
- cough
- shortness of breath
- fatigue
- muscle aches
- headache
- new loss of taste or smell
- sore throat
- runny nose
- nausea

---

[1] "Chikungunya," Centers for Disease Control and Prevention (CDC), November 28, 2023. Available online. URL: wwwnc.cdc.gov/travel/diseases/chikungunya. Accessed July 29, 2024.

- vomiting
- diarrhea

WHO IS AT RISK?
Coronavirus 2019 can affect anyone, but certain groups are more likely to develop severe illness, including older individuals, the immunocompromised, people with certain disabilities, or those with underlying health conditions. Protection measures such as vaccination, previous infection, and timely access to testing and treatment can mitigate the risk of severe illness.

TRAVEL CONSIDERATIONS FOR THOSE RECENTLY INFECTED
After ending isolation, you can travel, following the Centers for Disease Control and Prevention (CDC) guidelines, which may include testing and wearing a mask around others. If you are unable to wear a mask when around others, avoid public transportation, including airplanes, buses, and trains.

PREVENTING COVID-19 FOR TRAVELERS
To protect yourself and others while traveling:
- Ensure you are up-to-date with your COVID-19 vaccines.
- Wear masks in crowded or poorly ventilated indoor spaces, including public transportation and transportation hubs.
- Follow additional precautions if recently exposed to COVID-19.
- Do not travel while sick.

For those with weakened immune systems or increased risk of severe disease, consult with a health-care professional before deciding to travel. If you decide to travel, implement multiple prevention steps to enhance protection from COVID-19, even if vaccinated. These steps include improving ventilation, spending more time outdoors, avoiding contact with sick individuals, getting tested if symptoms develop, staying home if you suspect you have COVID-19, and seeking treatment if diagnosed.

Viral Infections

TESTING CONSIDERATIONS
Consider obtaining a COVID-19 test if you:
- develop symptoms before, during, or after travel
- plan to visit someone at high risk of severe illness from COVID-19
- were in high-risk exposure settings during travel, such as indoor crowded spaces without wearing a mask

IF YOU FEEL SICK AFTER TRAVELING
If you feel ill after traveling, especially with a fever, consult a health-care professional and inform them about your recent travel.[1]

Section 22.3 | Dengue Fever

WHAT IS DENGUE?
Dengue viruses are transmitted to humans through the bite of an infected mosquito. Typically, symptoms start within a few days of being bitten but can take up to two weeks to appear. These symptoms can be mild or severe and include fever accompanied by nausea, vomiting, rash, headache, eye pain, and joint and muscle pain. In severe cases, dengue can lead to shock, internal bleeding, and death. Not everyone infected with dengue will feel ill; only about one in four infected people develop symptoms. Those who have been infected previously are more likely to develop severe dengue, as are infants and pregnant women.

WHO IS AT RISK?
Mosquitoes that spread dengue primarily bite during the day and less frequently at night. They are prevalent in tropical and subtropical areas of the Americas, Africa, the Middle East, Asia, and the

---

[1] "COVID-19," Centers for Disease Control and Prevention (CDC), March 4, 2024. Available online. URL: wwwnc.cdc.gov/travel/diseases/covid19. Accessed July 29, 2024.

Pacific Islands. Travelers should check whether dengue is a concern at their destination. The risk of contracting dengue increases with:

- extensive outdoor exposure
- travel to regions with dengue risks during warm weather periods when mosquitoes are most active

PREVENTIVE MEASURES FOR TRAVELERS

To protect against dengue, travelers should take the following steps:

Use EPA-Registered Insect Repellent

- Choose repellents with active ingredients such as N,N-diethyl-meta-toluamide (DEET), picaridin, IR3535, oil of lemon eucalyptus (OLE), para-menthane-diol (PMD), or 2-undecanone. These ingredients are safe and effective, including for pregnant and breastfeeding women.
- Apply insect repellent after sunscreen.
- For children, use repellents safely by following label instructions, avoiding the use of OLE or PMD on those under three years, and not applying repellent to children's hands, eyes, mouth, or irritated skin. Adults should apply repellent to their hands and then apply it to the child's face.

Wear Protective Clothing

- Wear long-sleeved shirts and long pants.
- Treat clothing and gear with 0.5 percent permethrin or purchase permethrin-treated items. Permethrin-treated clothing remains protective through multiple washes.

Secure Accommodations

- Choose accommodations with air conditioning or protective screens on windows and doors.
- Use mosquito nets if sleeping outside or in unscreened rooms. Purchase nets that are compact, white, and rectangular, with at least 156 holes per square inch, and long enough to tuck under the mattress. Permethrin-treated nets offer added protection.

DENGUE VACCINE AND TRAVEL

Currently, there is no dengue vaccine recommended for travelers.

For further information on how to use permethrin safely and effectively, view the instructional video by the Centers for Disease Control and Prevention (CDC) at Permethrin-Treated Clothing and Gear (www.cdc.gov/mosquitoes/prevention/about-permethrin-treated-clothing-and-gear.html).

By adhering to these guidelines, travelers can significantly reduce their risk of contracting dengue while visiting areas where the virus is prevalent.[1]

Section 22.4 | Ebola and Marburg Diseases

WHAT ARE EBOLA AND MARBURG DISEASES?

Ebola disease and Marburg virus disease are classified as viral hemorrhagic fevers. These severe diseases harm organs and blood vessels and may lead to death. Infection with Ebola or Marburg viruses occurs through direct contact with:

- body fluids of an infected individual, whether alive or deceased, including blood, urine, saliva, sweat, feces, vomit, breast milk, and semen
- contaminated objects such as clothing, bedding, needles, and medical equipment that have been exposed to the body fluids of an infected person
- infected wild animals, such as bats and nonhuman primates, or their body fluids or meat (commonly called "bushmeat")

WHO IS AT RISK?

While most travelers have a low likelihood of exposure to Ebola or Marburg viruses, those traveling to sub-Saharan Africa, where

---

[1] "Dengue," Centers for Disease Control and Prevention (CDC), September 15, 2022. Available online. URL: wwwnc.cdc.gov/travel/diseases/dengue. Accessed July 29, 2024.

these viruses are prevalent, face increased risks. Specific risk factors include close interaction with or proximity to bats and nonhuman primates such as monkeys, chimpanzees, and gorillas. For instance, two tourists contracted the Marburg virus in 2008 in Uganda after visiting a bat-inhabited cave. Health-care workers caring for patients with Ebola or Marburg are also at heightened risk due to potential exposure to infected bodily fluids.

SYMPTOMS OF EBOLA AND MARBURG

The onset of symptoms for Ebola and Marburg can range from 2 to 21 days post-infection, with averages of 8 to 10 days for Ebola. Symptoms include sudden fever, chills, headaches, body aches, and a rash across the chest, back, and stomach. As the infection worsens, affected individuals may experience nausea, vomiting, chest pain, sore throat, abdominal pain, and diarrhea. Advanced stages of the diseases can lead to internal bleeding, critically low blood pressure (shock), multiple organ failure, and potentially death.

PREVENTIVE MEASURES FOR TRAVELERS

Travelers can reduce their risk of infection by adopting the following preventive measures:

- Avoid direct contact with ill individuals and any bodily fluids:
  - Refrain from physical affection such as kissing and hugging.
  - Do not use shared eating utensils or cups.
  - Avoid touching objects contaminated with bodily fluids.
- Exercise caution around animals:
  - Avoid contact with both live and deceased animals.
  - Steer clear of animal markets and farms.
  - Refrain from consuming or handling bushmeat.
  - Wear protective gear if your work involves contact with animals.

- Practice rigorous hand hygiene:
  - Frequently wash hands with soap and water, or use an alcohol-based hand sanitizer with at least 60 percent alcohol when soap and water are unavailable.
  - Avoid touching your face with unclean hands.
- Steer clear of contact with deceased individuals:
  - Avoid participating in funeral rituals involving direct contact with the deceased.
  - Do not touch objects that have come into contact with deceased individuals.

GUIDANCE AFTER TRAVEL

If you experience any symptoms, especially fever, after visiting regions affected by Ebola or Marburg outbreaks, promptly contact your local health department or a health-care provider. Inform them about your recent travel and symptoms. Isolate yourself from others to prevent potential spread.[1]

Section 22.5 | Hepatitis

HEPATITIS A
What Is Hepatitis A?

Hepatitis A virus (HAV) can cause liver disease. HAV is found in the stool and blood of infected people. People infected with HAV can spread it to others if you:

- eat food or drink beverages contaminated with HAV
- touch objects with the virus on them and then put your hands in your mouth
- have close, personal contact with an infected person, such as caring for them
- have sex with an infected person

---

[1] "Ebola and Marburg," Centers for Disease Control and Prevention (CDC), March 29, 2023. Available online. URL: wwwnc.cdc.gov/travel/diseases/ebola. Accessed July 29, 2024.

Who Is at Risk?

Hepatitis A is a common disease worldwide. Anyone who has not been vaccinated or previously infected can get hepatitis A. Travelers are more likely to get infected if they visit rural areas, travel in backcountry areas, or frequently eat or drink in settings of poor sanitation. However, infections can occur even in urban areas, resorts, or luxury hotels.

Symptoms of Hepatitis A

Symptoms may include:
- fever
- fatigue
- loss of appetite
- nausea
- vomiting
- abdominal pain
- dark urine
- diarrhea
- clay-colored bowel movements
- joint pain
- jaundice

Older children and adults who get hepatitis A feel sick for several weeks, but usually recover without lasting liver damage. Children younger than six usually do not have symptoms. In rare cases, hepatitis A can cause liver failure and death, especially in older individuals and those with other liver diseases.

Prevention for Travelers

Getting vaccinated is the best way to protect against hepatitis A. The vaccine is very effective and recommended for travelers six months of age or older going to countries where hepatitis A is common.[1]

---

[1] "Hepatitis A," Centers for Disease Control and Prevention (CDC), September 16, 2022. Available online. URL: wwwnc.cdc.gov/travel/diseases/hepatitis-a. Accessed July 29, 2024.

HEPATITIS B
What Is Hepatitis B?
Hepatitis B is a vaccine-preventable liver disease caused by the hepatitis B virus (HBV), found in the blood and body fluids of infected people. It spreads through:
- sexual contact with an infected partner
- sharing needles, syringes, or drug preparation equipment
- sharing personal items like razors or toothbrushes that might have come into contact with infected blood or body fluids
- direct contact with the blood or open sores of an infected person
- from mother to baby at birth

Who Is at Risk?
Hepatitis B occurs worldwide, especially in parts of Asia, Africa, South America, and the Caribbean. Travelers seeking medical care abroad are at higher risk.

Symptoms of Hepatitis B
Early symptoms may include:
- fever
- fatigue
- loss of appetite
- nausea
- vomiting
- abdominal pain
- dark urine
- clay-colored bowel movements
- joint pain
- jaundice

Chronic infection can lead to:
- liver failure
- cirrhosis
- liver cancer

Prevention for Travelers

The best way to protect yourself against hepatitis B is by getting vaccinated. The vaccine is usually given in three doses over six months.[2]

HEPATITIS C
What Is Hepatitis C?

Hepatitis C virus (HCV) can cause liver disease. Most people infected with HCV will have it for life, known as "chronic infection." It spreads through:

- sharing needles, syringes, or drug preparation equipment
- sharing personal care items that might have come into contact with infected blood
- unsterile tattoo, body piercing, or acupuncture equipment
- needlestick injuries in health-care settings
- having sex with an infected partner

Who Is at Risk?

Hepatitis C is common in parts of Asia and Africa. Travelers getting medical procedures, tattoos, or piercings abroad are at higher risk.

Symptoms of Hepatitis C

Many infected people have no symptoms. Those who do may experience:

- fever
- fatigue
- dark urine
- abdominal pain
- loss of appetite
- nausea
- vomiting

---

[2] "Hepatitis B," Centers for Disease Control and Prevention (CDC), November 8, 2022. Available online. URL: wwwnc.cdc.gov/travel/diseases/hepatitis-b. Accessed July 29, 2024.

- joint pain
- jaundice

Prevention for Travelers

There is no vaccine for hepatitis C. Prevent infection by avoiding risky behaviors and ensuring medical and dental equipment is sterilized.[3]

HEPATITIS E
What Is Hepatitis E?

Hepatitis E virus (HEV) can also cause liver disease. It is mainly found in areas with poor sanitation and spreads through contaminated food and water.

Who Is at Risk?

Hepatitis E is widespread in Asia and Africa. Travelers to regions with poor sanitation are at higher risk.

Symptoms of Hepatitis E

Symptoms may include:
- fever
- tiredness
- loss of appetite
- nausea
- vomiting
- stomach pain
- dark urine
- clay-colored bowel movements
- joint pain
- jaundice

Most people recover without lasting liver damage.

---

[3] "Hepatitis C," Centers for Disease Control and Prevention (CDC), September 16, 2022. Available online. URL: wwwnc.cdc.gov/travel/diseases/hepatitis-c. Accessed July 29, 2024.

Prevention for Travelers

There is no approved vaccine in the United States. Prevent infection by choosing food and drinks carefully, avoiding unclean water, and ensuring food is thoroughly cooked.[4]

Section 22.6 | Human Immunodeficiency Virus (HIV)

WHAT IS HUMAN IMMUNODEFICIENCY VIRUS?

Human immunodeficiency virus (HIV) targets the immune system and is transmitted through certain body fluids, including blood, sexual fluids (such as semen, vaginal, or rectal fluids), and breast milk. The primary modes of transmission are unprotected sexual intercourse (vaginal or anal) with an infected person and sharing needles or other drug injection equipment.

SYMPTOMS OF HUMAN IMMUNODEFICIENCY VIRUS

Initial symptoms of HIV may include cough, body aches, headaches, nasal congestion, and sore throat, often resembling flu-like illnesses. These symptoms may resolve independently, leading some to overlook them. Notably, some individuals may exhibit no early symptoms and feel healthy. Testing is the only definitive method to determine HIV status.

Over time, HIV compromises the immune system, increasing susceptibility to various diseases, such as heart disease, kidney disease, liver disease, and cancer. If untreated, HIV progresses to acquired immune deficiency syndrome (AIDS), the most critical phase of the infection. Individuals with AIDS are prone to severe opportunistic infections (OIs) that do not normally affect healthy people, often leading to death. Although no cure exists, timely diagnosis and appropriate medical care can manage and control HIV effectively.

---

[4] "Hepatitis E," Centers for Disease Control and Prevention (CDC), September 21, 2022. Available online. URL: wwwnc.cdc.gov/travel/diseases/hepatitis-e. Accessed July 29, 2024.

WHO IS AT RISK?

Travelers generally face a low risk of contracting HIV unless they participate in high-risk behaviors, such as unprotected sex or needle sharing.

Health-care workers and travelers receiving medical care in regions with inadequate blood screening or sterilization practices, particularly in low-income countries, are at a heightened risk of HIV from contaminated needles or medical equipment.

Globally, HIV affects diverse populations, with sub-Saharan Africa experiencing the most significant burden. However, other regions, including Asia and the Pacific, Latin America, the Caribbean, Eastern Europe, and Central Asia, also report substantial HIV prevalence.

PREVENTATIVE MEASURES FOR TRAVELERS

- Discuss pre-exposure prophylaxis (PrEP) with your health-care provider; which is available as a pill or injection and is most effective when prescribed.
- Before engaging in sexual relations with a new partner, discuss your sexual and drug-use histories, disclose your HIV status, and undergo testing for HIV and other sexually transmitted infections (STIs).
- Consistently use condoms correctly during all sexual activities, including vaginal, oral, or anal intercourse.
- Avoid drug injection or sharing of needles. If drug injection is unavoidable, use only new, sterile syringes and needles.
- Ensure new, sterile needles are used for tattoos, piercings, or acupuncture performed abroad.
- Verify that medical or dental equipment abroad is unused or properly sterilized.
- If you are HIV-positive and traveling, carry sufficient medication for your entire trip as availability may vary by country.
- Consult with a doctor or travel medicine specialist at least four weeks before travel to discuss vaccine eligibility and necessary precautions.

Understanding and preventing HIV infection is crucial for maintaining health, especially when traveling. By taking proactive measures such as discussing PrEP, using condoms, and ensuring medical equipment is sterile, travelers can significantly reduce their risk of HIV infection. Awareness and preparedness are key to safeguarding health in global settings.[1]

Section 22.7 | Influenza

Getting vaccinated each year is the best way to reduce the risk of flu and its potential complications. Depending on your destination, you may need a flu vaccine at other times of the year before traveling.

FLU SEASON BY REGION

- **Northern Hemisphere.** Flu season can start as early as October and last until April or May.
- **Temperate Southern Hemisphere.** In regions with distinct seasons, flu activity typically occurs from April to September.
- **Tropics.** Flu activity occurs throughout the year.

VACCINATION RECOMMENDATIONS

Travelers in large tourist groups, such as on cruise ships, where they interact with people from various parts of the world, may be at an increased risk. It is advisable to get vaccinated at least two weeks before travel because it takes that long for immunity to develop after vaccination. Vaccination is particularly crucial for individuals at higher risk of severe flu complications. If you have already received your annual flu vaccine, you usually do not need to be vaccinated again during the same season.

---

[1] "HIV," Centers for Disease Control and Prevention (CDC), October 19, 2022. Available online. URL: wwwnc.cdc. gov/travel/diseases/hiv. Accessed July 29, 2024.

TRAVEL RESTRICTIONS IF SICK

Do not travel if you are sick with flu-like symptoms. Stay home until you are fever-free for at least 24 hours without the use of fever-reducing medicine, such as acetaminophen. Symptoms of the flu include:

- cough or sore throat
- runny or stuffy nose
- muscle or body aches
- headache
- fatigue
- in some cases, fever
- vomiting and diarrhea (more common in children)

DURING TRAVEL

While traveling, adhere to local guidelines and practice healthy habits:

- Avoid close contact with sick individuals.
- Wash your hands frequently with soap and running water, especially after coughing or sneezing.
- If soap and water are not available, use a hand sanitizer containing at least 60-percent alcohol. Ensure you cover all surfaces of your hands and rub them together until they feel dry.
- When you cough or sneeze, cover your mouth and nose with a tissue and dispose of the used tissue in a trash can. If a tissue is unavailable, cough or sneeze into your upper sleeve, not your hands.

WHAT TO DO IF YOU FEEL SICK

Most people with the flu will recover without needing medical care. However, if you experience severe illness or are at risk of serious flu complications, seek medical attention immediately.

A U.S. consular officer can assist you in finding local medical care in a foreign country. To contact a U.S. Embassy or Consulate, call Overseas Citizens Services at 888-407-4747 from the United States or Canada, or 00-1-202-501-4444 from other countries. Additionally, you can visit the websites of U.S. Embassies,

Consulates, and Diplomatic missions for contact information for the local U.S. Embassy in the country you are visiting. Always follow all local health recommendations.[1]

Section 22.8 | Norovirus

WHAT IS NOROVIRUS?

Norovirus, belonging to the genus Norovirus, is a nonenveloped, single-stranded ribonucleic acid (RNA) virus. Previously known as "Norwalk-like viruses," "Norwalk viruses," and "small round-structured viruses," norovirus is a primary cause of viral gastroenteritis. It is often misattributed as "stomach flu," despite no biological connection to influenza viruses.

TRANSMISSION OF NOROVIRUS

Transmission primarily occurs through the fecal-oral route, either directly from person to person or indirectly via contaminated food or water. It can also spread through fomites and aerosols containing vomit particles.

EPIDEMIOLOGY OF NOROVIRUS

Norovirus outbreaks are common in close-quarter settings such as cruise ships, camps, dormitories, and hotels, where rapid transmission is facilitated. It frequently contaminates ready-to-eat cold foods like salads and sandwiches, and raw shellfish, particularly oysters, due to their ability to concentrate viral particles from water. Ice contamination has also been implicated in outbreaks. Environmental contamination, such as on cruise ships, can lead to successive outbreaks among new passengers. Reports also exist of norovirus transmission on airplanes, likely through contaminated lavatories or symptomatic passengers.

---

[1] "Flu (Influenza)," Centers for Disease Control and Prevention (CDC), November 14, 2022. Available online. URL: wwwnc.cdc.gov/travel/diseases/influenza-seasonal-zoonotic-and-pandemic. Accessed July 29, 2024.

Globally, most children will contract norovirus at least once by age five. The virus is omnipresent year-round, peaking in winter in temperate regions. It causes approximately 18 percent of all acute gastroenteritis cases worldwide, potentially leading to around 200,000 deaths annually. In the United States, it is the leading cause of medically attended gastroenteritis in young children and accounts for about 50 percent of all foodborne disease outbreaks, causing roughly 19–21 million illnesses annually.

CLINICAL PRESENTATION OF NOROVIRUS
Symptoms typically include acute vomiting, nonbloody diarrhea, abdominal cramps, nausea, and sometimes a low-grade fever, appearing 12–48 hours after exposure. Although the illness is generally brief, lasting one to three days, severe dehydration can occur, especially in the very young or elderly, necessitating medical attention.

DIAGNOSIS OF NOROVIRUS INFECTION
Diagnosis is mainly based on symptoms as routine diagnostic testing to guide clinical management is uncommon. However, during outbreaks, laboratory testing like real-time reverse-transcription quantitative PCR (RT-qPCR) is utilized to identify disease clusters. The Centers for Disease Control and Prevention (CDC) recommends contacting local health departments for outbreak investigations.

TREATMENT OF NOROVIRUS INFECTION
Treatment is primarily supportive, focusing on oral or intravenous rehydration. Antidiarrheals and antiemetics are generally not recommended for children. In adults, antiemetic, antimotility, and antisecretory agents can support rehydration. Antibiotics are ineffective against norovirus.

PREVENTION OF NOROVIRUS INFECTION
While there is currently no vaccine for norovirus, development is underway. Prevention strategies include rigorous handwashing with soap and water for at least 20 seconds and using alcohol-based

hand sanitizers only as a supplementary measure. Travelers should also practice diligent cleanliness, including disinfecting contaminated surfaces with EPA-approved products or a dilute bleach solution and washing soiled clothing in hot water. To control the spread of the virus, isolated measures are advisable for affected individuals on cruise ships and in institutional settings like hospitals, long-term care facilities, and schools.

Norovirus remains a significant global health challenge, particularly in environments where close contact is unavoidable. Continued emphasis on hygiene and isolation during outbreaks is crucial in mitigating its effect.[1]

Section 22.9 | West Nile Virus

WHAT IS WEST NILE VIRUS?

West Nile virus (WNV) is primarily transmitted to humans through the bite of an infected mosquito. Although rare, there have been instances of transmission via blood transfusion, organ donation, and from mother to child during pregnancy, childbirth, or breastfeeding.

SYMPTOMS OF WEST NILE VIRUS

Most individuals infected with WNV do not exhibit symptoms. Those who do may experience:

- fever
- headache
- tiredness
- nausea
- vomiting
- muscle aches
- a rash, typically lasting a few days to several weeks

---

[1] "Norovirus," Centers for Disease Control and Prevention (CDC), May 1, 2023. Available online. URL: wwwnc.cdc.gov/travel/yellowbook/2024/infections-diseases/norovirus. Accessed July 29, 2024.

Severe cases are more common in adults over 60 or those with specific medical conditions, presenting symptoms such as:
- high fever
- headache
- neck stiffness
- disorientation
- coma
- tremors
- convulsions
- muscle weakness
- vision loss
- numbness
- paralysis

WHO IS AT RISK?

West Nile virus is found globally, with potential exposure for travelers to Africa, Europe, the Middle East, west and Central Asia, and North America. Risks are elevated for those spending significant time outdoors or traveling during peak mosquito seasons, particularly in the summer.

PREVENTING WEST NILE VIRUS

Currently, no vaccines or medications prevent WNV. The primary prevention strategy is mosquito bite avoidance.

EFFECTIVE MOSQUITO PREVENTION STRATEGIES

- **Use insect repellents.** Choose repellents with active ingredients such as N,N-diethyl-meta-toluamide (DEET), picaridin, IR3535, oil of lemon eucalyptus (OLE), para-menthane-diol (PMD), or 2-undecanone. Use the U.S. Environmental Protection Agency's (EPA) search tool at www.epa.gov/insect-repellents/find-repellent-right-you to find suitable products. Apply repellent after sunscreen and follow label instructions carefully.
- **Safety for children and babies.** Dress children in long sleeves and pants, use mosquito netting over strollers and

carriers, and adhere to guidelines regarding repellent use on young children, particularly avoiding OLE or PMD for those under three years old.

- **Wear protective clothing.** Long-sleeved shirts and long pants can provide additional protection. Treat clothing and gear with 0.5 percent permethrin, which can be effective through multiple washes. Avoid direct application of permethrin on the skin.
- **Secure your living area**. Opt for accommodations with air conditioning or protective screens on windows and doors. Use mosquito nets if sleeping outside or in unscreened rooms. Preferably, use permethrin-treated nets for enhanced protection.
- **Post-bite care**. If bitten, avoid scratching and apply over-the-counter (OTC) anti-itch or antihistamine cream to alleviate itching.

For more details on using permethrin and mosquito nets, visit www.cdc.gov/mosquitoes/mosquito-bites/how-to-use-permethrin.html. Travelers especially should be vigilant about mosquito bite prevention, a critical step in avoiding WNV and maintaining health during travel.[1]

Section 22.10 | Yellow Fever

WHAT IS YELLOW FEVER?

Yellow fever is a severe disease caused by the yellow fever virus. Most individuals infected with the virus do not experience symptoms or only have mild ones. However, symptoms such as fever, chills, headache, backache, and muscle aches can develop three to six days after infection. Approximately, 12 percent of symptomatic

---

[1] "West Nile Virus," Centers for Disease Control and Prevention (CDC), September 27, 2022. Available online. URL: wwwnc.cdc.gov/travel/diseases/west-nile-virus. Accessed April 4, 2024.

individuals may develop serious conditions, including jaundice, bleeding, shock, organ failure, and potentially death.

WHO IS AT RISK?
The yellow fever virus is transmitted by mosquitoes found in certain parts of South America and Africa. Travelers to these regions are at risk of infection.

WHAT CAN TRAVELERS DO TO PROTECT THEMSELVES?
To safeguard against yellow fever, travelers should get vaccinated and take measures to prevent mosquito bites.

Yellow Fever Vaccine: Requirements and Recommendations
Some countries require travelers to provide proof of yellow fever vaccination as a public health measure to prevent the importation of the virus. These requirements can apply to all or some travelers, and the Centers for Disease Control and Prevention (CDC) does not influence these regulations.

Independently, the CDC recommends yellow fever vaccinations for travelers to countries with a risk of the virus. These recommendations aim to prevent infection during travel.

GETTING VACCINATED
Travelers should visit a yellow fever vaccination clinic to verify if vaccination is necessary for their destination. It is advised to get the vaccine at least 10 days before travel, as immunity to the virus takes this time to develop. While a single dose offers lifetime protection for most people, a booster dose after 10 years may be recommended for certain travelers. Discuss your medical history with your health-care provider to understand any risks, especially if you are over 60 years of age, immunocompromised, pregnant, or nursing.

PROOF OF VACCINATION
Upon vaccination, you will receive the International Certificate of Vaccination or Prophylaxis (ICVP; also known as the "yellow card"),

which serves as proof of vaccination. You must present the original signed and stamped ICVP along with your passport to immigration officials in countries that require proof of vaccination.

Preventing Mosquito Bites

To prevent mosquito bites, use an U.S. Environmental Protection Agency (EPA)-registered insect repellent containing one of the following active ingredients: N,N-diethyl-meta-toluamide (DEET), picaridin, IR3535, oil of lemon eucalyptus (OLE), para-menthane-diol (PMD), or 2-undecanone. Use EPA's search tool to select the right product (www.epa.gov/insect-repellents/find-repellent-right-you).

TIPS FOR USING INSECT REPELLENT ON BABIES AND CHILDREN

- Dress children in clothing that covers their arms and legs.
- Cover strollers and baby carriers with mosquito netting.
- Follow the label instructions when applying repellent. Avoid using products with OLE or PMD on children under three years old.
- Do not apply repellent to children's hands, eyes, mouth, or irritated skin. Apply it to your hands first, then to the child's face.

CLOTHING AND GEAR TREATMENT

Use 0.5 percent permethrin to treat clothing and gear like boots, pants, socks, and tents, or purchase permethrin-treated items. Permethrin is an insecticide that remains effective after multiple washes. Follow product instructions for application and do not apply directly to the skin.

Accommodation Tips

Choose accommodations with air conditioning or protective screens on windows and doors. If these are not available, use a mosquito net, especially when sleeping outdoors or in unscreened rooms.

Preventing yellow fever starts with vaccination and includes diligent efforts to avoid mosquito bites. Understanding the risks and preparedness strategies is crucial for anyone traveling to regions where yellow fever is endemic. By taking these proactive steps, travelers can significantly reduce their risk of contracting this potentially deadly virus.[1]

Section 22.11 | Zika

WHAT IS ZIKA VIRUS?
Zika virus is primarily transmitted through the bite of an infected mosquito. It can also spread through blood transfusions, organ donations, and from mother to child during pregnancy, childbirth, or breastfeeding. While many infected individuals do not exhibit symptoms or experience only mild effects, outbreaks of the Zika virus can occur globally.

HOW ZIKA VIRUS SPREADS
Zika virus can spread in several ways:
- **Mosquito bites**. Infected mosquitoes transmit the virus to people.
- **From mother to child**. Transmission can occur during pregnancy or at birth.
- **Sexual contact**. Zika can be passed through sexual activity, remaining in semen longer than in other body fluids.

PREVENTING ZIKA VIRUS FOR TRAVELERS
- **Pregnant women**. Avoid travel to areas with Zika outbreaks due to the risk of serious birth defects.

---

[1] "Yellow Fever," Centers for Disease Control and Prevention (CDC), July 6, 2023. Available online. URL: wwwnc. cdc.gov/travel/diseases/yellow-fever. Accessed July 29, 2024.

- **Pretravel consultation.** Those considering pregnancy or traveling to areas with Zika risk should consult health-care providers to discuss the risks and necessary precautions.
- **Mosquito bite prevention.** All travelers should use EPA-registered insect repellents with ingredients such as N,N-diethyl-meta-toluamide (DEET), picaridin, or oil of lemon eucalyptus (OLE). Wear long-sleeved shirts and pants, and stay in places with air conditioning or adequate window and door screens.
- **Sexual transmission.** Use condoms or abstain from sex to prevent Zika transmission, especially important for those pregnant or planning pregnancy.

SPECIAL PRECAUTIONS

- **Pregnant women.** Should not travel to areas with known Zika outbreaks and discuss any travel plans to areas with potential risk with their health-care provider.
- **Partners of pregnant women.** Should use condoms or abstain from sex for the duration of the pregnancy if exposed to Zika.
- **Those considering pregnancy.** Couples should wait three months after returning from travel before trying to conceive if the man traveled, and two months if the woman traveled.

DURING TRAVEL: PROTECT YOURSELF

- **Use insect repellents.** The U.S. Environmental Protection Agency (EPA)-registered insect repellents with active ingredients such as DEET, picaridin, IR3535, OLE, para-menthane-diol (PMD), or 2-undecanone shall be used.
- **Cover exposed skin.** Wear long-sleeved shirts and long pants.
- **Accommodations.** Stay in places with air conditioning and screens, or use a mosquito bed net.
- **Remove standing water.** Take measures to control mosquitoes inside and outside during extended stays.

AFTER TRAVEL: PROTECT OTHERS

- **Mosquito bite prevention**. Continue using mosquito repellent for three weeks to prevent spreading the virus to uninfected mosquitoes.
- **Prevent sexual transmission**. Use condoms or abstain from sex for at least three months if you are a man and two months if you are a woman to prevent passing the virus to partners.

IF YOU SUSPECT ZIKA INFECTION

- **Seek medical advice**. Consult a health-care provider if you develop symptoms such as fever, rash, joint pain, or red eyes.
- **Safe medication use**. For symptoms, take acetaminophen, but avoid aspirin and non-steroidal anti-inflammatory drugs (NSAIDs) until a health-care provider rules out dengue.
- **Testing**. A blood or urine test can confirm a Zika infection.

While there is currently no vaccine or specific treatment for the Zika virus, understanding the modes of transmission and taking appropriate preventive measures can significantly reduce the risk of its infection.[1]

---

[1] "Zika," Centers for Disease Control and Prevention (CDC), October 19, 2022. Available online. URL: wwwnc.cdc.gov/travel/diseases/zika. Accessed July 29, 2024.

Chapter 23 | Fungal and Parasitic Infections

Chapter Contents

Section 23.1 | Histoplasmosis

WHAT IS HISTOPLASMOSIS?
Histoplasmosis is caused by *Histoplasma capsulatum*, a thermal-dimorphic fungus that grows as a mold in the environment and as a yeast within animal and human hosts.

TRANSMISSION OF HISTOPLASMOSIS
The disease is transmitted through inhaling spores from the environment, particularly from soil contaminated with bat guano or bird droppings. It does not transmit from person to person.

EPIDEMIOLOGY OF HISTOPLASMOSIS
The global epidemiology of histoplasmosis is not fully understood, and cases among travelers are likely underreported. At-risk groups include adventure tourists, humanitarian aid workers, long-term travelers and expatriates, study-abroad students, and individuals visiting friends and relatives. Engaging in activities that disturb soil, especially in areas frequented by bats and birds, increases the risk of histoplasmosis. The disease also affects immigrants from endemic areas who become immunocompromised.

CLINICAL PRESENTATION
The incubation period ranges from 3 to 17 days. While about 90 percent of infections are asymptomatic or mild, acute pulmonary histoplasmosis can cause symptoms such as body aches, chest pain, chills, cough, fatigue, fever, and headache. Most individuals recover spontaneously within weeks, though fatigue may linger. High-dose exposures can result in severe disease, and dissemination to organs such as the central nervous system (CNS) and gastrointestinal tract is possible in immunocompromised individuals. Misdiagnosis as other diseases, such as tuberculosis, is common in regions where both pathogens are endemic.

DIAGNOSIS OF HISTOPLASMOSIS

Diagnostic methods include culture and histopathologic identification, with antigen and antibody testing providing additional tools, particularly for travel-associated cases. The Centers for Disease Control and Prevention's (CDC) Mycotic Diseases Branch (www. cdc.gov/fungal/hcp/laboratories/index.html) offers diagnostic support through immunodiagnostics and molecular testing.

TREATMENT OF HISTOPLASMOSIS

Treatment is generally not required for immunocompetent individuals with acute, localized pulmonary infections. For more severe cases, or symptoms persisting over a month, antifungal treatments such as azole drugs or amphotericin B are recommended. Steroids may also be beneficial for patients with acute respiratory distress.

PREVENTION OF HISTOPLASMOSIS

High-risk individuals should avoid areas such as bat-inhabited caves. While no vaccine exists, chemoprophylaxis with itraconazole is advised for certain immunocompromised individuals, including those living with human immunodeficiency virus (HIV).

Understanding and managing histoplasmosis requires awareness of its transmission, clinical manifestations, and prevention strategies, particularly for individuals traveling to or residing in endemic regions.[1]

Section 23.2 | Valley Fever (Coccidioidomycosis)

Valley fever (coccidioidomycosis) is caused by the fungi: *Coccidioides immitis* and *Coccidioides posadasii*.

---

[1] "Histoplasmosis," Centers for Disease Control and Prevention (CDC), May 1, 2023. Available online. URL: wwwnc. cdc.gov/travel/yellowbook/2024/infections-diseases/histoplasmosis. Accessed July 29, 2024.

TRANSMISSION OF COCCIDIOIDOMYCOSIS

This infection is transmitted through inhalation of fungal conidia from the environment. Direct person-to-person transmission does not occur.

EPIDEMIOLOGY

Coccidioides is endemic to the western United States, particularly Arizona and Southern California, and parts of Mexico and Central and South America. Groups at increased risk include adventure tourists, expatriates, humanitarian aid workers, long-term travelers, and travelers visiting friends and relatives (VFRs). Risk is heightened by activities that disturb the soil or generate outdoor dust, such as community house-building, gardening, four-wheeling, and horseback riding. Outbreaks have also been linked to archaeological digs, construction, and military exercises.

CLINICAL PRESENTATION

The incubation period for coccidioidomycosis ranges from 7 to 21 days. Approximately, 40 percent of those exposed develop symptoms, which can vary from mild pulmonary issues to severe disseminated disease. Common symptoms include cough, persistent fatigue, and occasionally fever. Other possible symptoms are shortness of breath, headache, joint pain, muscle aches, night sweats, and rash. While many infections resolve within weeks to months, severe cases may result in chronic lung disease or dissemination to the central nervous system, bones, joints, or skin, sometimes requiring lifelong treatment.

DIAGNOSIS OF COCCIDIOIDOMYCOSIS

As a nationally notifiable disease in the United States, coccidioidomycosis is diagnosed through methods such as culture, histopathology, molecular techniques, and serology. Isolating *Coccidioides* in culture provides a definitive diagnosis. Molecular techniques such as DNA probes and polymerase chain reaction (PCR) testing, along with enzyme immunoassays (EIA) for antibody detection, enhance diagnostic accuracy.

TREATMENT FOR COCCIDIOIDOMYCOSIS

Management of uncomplicated primary pulmonary coccidioidomycosis varies. Some experts suggest no treatment for mild cases, while others recommend antifungal therapy to mitigate symptoms. High-risk patients, or those showing signs of severe pulmonary or disseminated disease, should receive antifungal treatment. Options include amphotericin B and azole antifungals like fluconazole or itraconazole.

PREVENTION OF COCCIDIOIDOMYCOSIS

Travelers to endemic areas should minimize exposure to dust. Protective measures include using N95 respirators, staying indoors during dust storms, and avoiding soil-disturbing activities. Indoor air filtration and prophylactic antifungal medications are additional preventive strategies recommended under certain conditions.

Awareness and preventive measures are crucial for travelers and residents in endemic regions to reduce the risk of contracting coccidioidomycosis, especially for those engaging in high-risk activities.[1]

Section 23.3 | Giardiasis

WHAT IS GIARDIASIS?

Giardiasis is an illness caused by the anaerobic protozoan parasite *Giardia duodenalis* (*Giardia lamblia* or *Giardia intestinalis*).

TRANSMISSION OF GIARDIASIS

Giardia is transmitted through the fecal-oral route. Characteristics such as a low infectious dose, protracted communicability, and moderate chlorine tolerance make it well-suited for transmission

---

[1] "Coccidioidomycosis/Valley Fever," Centers for Disease Control and Prevention (CDC), May 1, 2023. Available online. URL: wwwnc.cdc.gov/travel/yellowbook/2024/infections-diseases/coccidioidomycosis-valley-fever. Accessed July 29, 2024.

via contaminated drinking and recreational water. Additional transmission routes include direct contact with feces during patient care, sexual activity, consumption of contaminated food, or contact with fecally contaminated surfaces.

EPIDEMIOLOGY

Giardia is endemic worldwide, including in the United States. According to data from the GeoSentinel Global Surveillance Network from 2000 to 2012, it is a leading cause of acute diarrhea among U.S. travelers returning from various global regions. Risk factors include prolonged travel in areas with poor sanitation and consuming untreated water from natural sources. It is also commonly found in refugees and internationally adopted children, many of whom are asymptomatic.

CLINICAL PRESENTATION

While many infected individuals are asymptomatic, symptomatic cases typically develop one to two weeks after exposure and resolve within two to four weeks. Symptoms include abdominal cramps, anorexia, bloating, diarrhea with foul-smelling, greasy stools, flatulence, and nausea. Other potential symptoms include the gradual onset of loose stools, fatigue, and sometimes prominent upper gastrointestinal symptoms. Fever and vomiting are rare. Chronic conditions such as reactive arthritis and irritable bowel syndrome can occur post-infection. In children, severe infections can lead to developmental delays and stunted growth.

DIAGNOSIS OF GIARDIASIS

Diagnosing giardiasis involves detecting *Giardia* cysts or trophozoites in stool, which can be elusive. Employing less than or equal to three stool specimens over several days can improve diagnostic sensitivity. Techniques include direct fluorescent antibody testing (considered the gold standard), microscopy with trichrome staining, enzyme immunoassays, rapid immunochromatographic assays, and molecular assays. Only molecular testing can accurately identify specific genotypes and subtypes of *Giardia*. Retesting may be necessary if symptoms persist after treatment.

TREATMENT OF GIARDIASIS

Effective treatments include metronidazole, tinidazole, and nitazoxanide, with alternatives such as furazolidone, paromomycin, and quinacrine. Due to diagnostic challenges, empiric treatment is often utilized for patients with typical symptoms and relevant exposure history.

PREVENTION OF GIARDIASIS

Preventive measures include adhering to safe water precautions, practicing good hygiene, and avoiding potentially contaminated water. Travelers should ensure water safety by using commercially bottled water or treating water when necessary. Avoidance of water ingestion during recreational activities and meticulous handwashing are crucial for preventing infection.[1]

Section 23.4 | Leishmaniasis

WHAT IS LEISHMANIASIS?

Leishmaniasis is a parasitic disease caused by an infection with *Leishmania* parasites, which are spread by the bite of infected sand flies. Leishmaniasis is classified as a neglected tropical disease (NTD).

FORMS

There are several forms of leishmaniasis in people:
- **Cutaneous leishmaniasis (CL).** The most common form, which causes skin sores.

---

[1] "Giardiasis," Centers for Disease Control and Prevention (CDC), May 1, 2023. Available online. URL: wwwnc.cdc.gov/travel/yellowbook/2024/infections-diseases/giardiasis. Accessed July 29, 2024.

- **Mucosal leishmaniasis (ML).** A severe type of CL that can cause sores in the nose, mouth, or throat and can be life-threatening.
- **Visceral leishmaniasis (VL).** A less common form, especially in the United States, which affects internal organs. If untreated, severe cases of VL can be deadly.

SIGNS AND SYMPTOMS

Signs and symptoms vary based on the form of leishmaniasis. People may or may not experience signs and symptoms.

- **CL.** Those who develop symptoms have one or more skin sores, which can change in size and appearance over time. The skin sores usually develop within a few weeks or months of the sand fly bite and are often painless.
- **ML.** It is a form of leishmaniasis that affects the mucous membranes (most commonly the nose, but also the mouth and throat). ML can result from infection with some types of parasites that cause CL in parts of Central and South America and, rarely, other places.
- **VL.** A few *Leishmania* species cause VL. People with VL may develop fever, generalized illness, and anemia (low red blood cells). VL often affects internal organs (especially the spleen, liver, and bone marrow) and can be life-threatening. People with VL usually become sick within months (though it can be years) of the sand fly bite. If untreated, VL is typically deadly.

WHO IS AT RISK?

Anyone who lives in or travels to an area where *Leishmania* parasites occur and is bitten by an infected sand fly is at risk for leishmaniasis. It is more common in rural areas but can also occur on the outskirts of some cities. People are most likely to be bitten from dusk to dawn. Leishmaniasis occurs in parts of approximately 90 countries, usually in tropical or subtropical climates.

Places with Increased Risk

Leishmaniasis occurs in approximately 90 countries in the tropics, subtropics, and southern Europe. The ecological settings range from rain forests to deserts. It is usually more common in rural areas than in urban areas, though it is found on the outskirts of some cities. Climate and other environmental variations can potentially expand the geographic range of sand fly vectors and, thus, areas of the world where leishmaniasis occurs.

In the Eastern Hemisphere, leishmaniasis occurs in parts of Asia, the Middle East, Africa (particularly in Northeastern Africa, with some cases elsewhere), and Southern Europe. In the Western Hemisphere, leishmaniasis occurs in parts of Mexico, Central America, South America, and the southwestern United States. Leishmaniasis is not found in Australia, the Pacific Islands, Chile, or Uruguay.

Leishmaniasis in the United States

Most cases of leishmaniasis diagnosed in the US are in people who were infected while traveling or living in other countries. Occasionally, people have had locally acquired CL, especially in Texas and rarely in other states (e.g., Oklahoma and Arizona). There have been no known cases of acquired VL in the United States.

HOW IT SPREADS

The main way people get infected with leishmaniasis is through the bite of an infected female sand fly. People may not notice the bites because sand flies are silent and very small, and the bites can be painless for many people. On average, sand flies that transmit the parasite are only about one-fourth the size of mosquitoes (sometimes even smaller). Sand flies are usually most active at twilight, evening, and nighttime hours (dusk to dawn).

Some species of *Leishmania* parasites can also be spread via contaminated needles (needle sharing) or blood transfusions. There have also been reports of congenital transmission (mother passing an infection to her baby during pregnancy or at birth).

PREVENTION

There are no vaccines or drugs to prevent leishmaniasis. The best way to prevent infection is to protect yourself from sand fly bites through preventive measures. Even if you have already had leishmaniasis, it is possible to get it again. People can take the following preventive measures:

- **When indoors.** Stay in safe indoor areas (e.g., well-screened or air-conditioned areas). Be aware that sand flies are much smaller than mosquitoes and can get through smaller holes. Spray living and sleeping areas with insecticide to kill insects. If you are not sleeping in a well-screened or air-conditioned area, use a small mesh bed net and tuck it under your mattress. If possible, use an insecticide-treated bed net. Screens, curtains, sheets, and clothing can also be treated with insecticide. Clothing should be re-treated after five washes.
- **When outdoors.** When possible, wear clothing to minimize the amount of skin you have exposed (e.g., long-sleeved shirts, long pants, socks; tuck your shirt into your pants). Use U.S. Environmental Protection Agency (EPA)-registered insect repellent on exposed skin and under the ends of sleeves and pant legs. Repellents that contain N,N-diethyl-meta-toluamide (DEET) are generally the most effective.

DIAGNOSIS

If you have traveled or lived in a part of the world where leishmaniasis occurs and have symptoms, talk to your health-care provider. The staff of the Centers for Disease Control and Prevention (CDC) can advise your health-care provider and help with laboratory testing for leishmaniasis. Your health-care provider will test tissue samples from skin sores (for CL) or from bone marrow (for VL) to examine for diagnosis. Blood tests can be helpful for VL.

TREATMENT AND RECOVERY

The Centers for Disease Control and Prevention (CDC) staff can advise your health-care provider on whether your case of leishmaniasis should be treated and, if so, with what type of treatment.

- **CL.** Different types of treatment are available for CL, and the choice of treatment depends on multiple factors, including the species of *Leishmania* parasite involved. In some cases, skin sores from CL might heal on their own without treatment depending on the species involved. *Leishmania* skin sores can take months to years to heal and can leave significant scars.
- **ML.** Proper treatment is important for the *Leishmania* species that cause ML to prevent mucosal tissue destruction in the nose, mouth, or throat. Without treatment, ML can be life-threatening if it affects the throat.
- **VL.** It is important to recognize and treat VL early. If not treated, severe (advanced) cases of VL are typically deadly. In people with compromised immune systems (e.g., HIV, malnutrition), VL can be difficult to treat.[1]

Section 23.5 | Malaria

WHAT IS MALARIA?

Malaria is a disease caused by a parasite. Mosquitoes spread the parasite to people when they bite them. Symptoms usually appear within 7–30 days but can take up to one year to develop. They may include high fevers, shaking chills, and flu-like illness. Without treatment, malaria can cause severe illness and death.

WHO IS AT RISK?

The mosquitoes that spread malaria are found in Africa, Central and South America, parts of the Caribbean, Asia, Eastern Europe,

---

[1] "About Leishmaniasis," Centers for Disease Control and Prevention (CDC), March 11, 2024. Available online. URL: www.cdc.gov/leishmaniasis/about. Accessed July 29, 2024.

and the South Pacific. Travelers going to these countries may get bitten by mosquitoes and become infected. About 2,000 cases of malaria are diagnosed in the United States annually, mostly among returned travelers.

WHAT CAN TRAVELERS DO TO PREVENT MALARIA?

Travelers can protect themselves from malaria by taking prescription medicine and preventing mosquito bites. There is no malaria vaccine.

Take Malaria Medicine

Check your destination to see if you should take prescription malaria medication. Depending on the medicine you take, you will need to start taking this medicine multiple days before your trip, as well as during and after your trip. Talk to your doctor about which medicine you should take.

Use an Insect Repellent

Use U.S. Environmental Protection Agency (EPA)-registered insect repellents with one of the following active ingredients. When used as directed, EPA-registered insect repellents are proven safe and effective, even for pregnant and breastfeeding women. If you are also using sunscreen, always apply insect repellent after sunscreen.

- N, N-diethyl-meta-toluamide or diethyltoluamide (DEET)
- picaridin (known as "KBR 3023" and "icaridin" outside the United States)
- IR3535
- oil of lemon eucalyptus (OLE)
- para-menthane-diol (PMD)
- 2-undecanone

Find the right insect repellent for you by using the EPA's search tool (www.epa.gov/insect-repellents/find-repellent-right-you).

INSECT REPELLENT TIPS FOR BABIES AND CHILDREN

- Dress your child in clothing that covers arms and legs.
- Cover strollers and baby carriers with mosquito netting.
- When using insect repellent on your child:
  - Always follow label instructions.
  - Do not use products containing OLE or PMD on children under three years old.
  - Do not apply insect repellent to a child's hands, eyes, mouth, cuts, or irritated skin.
  - Adults should spray insect repellent onto their hands and then apply it to the child's face.
  - If also using sunscreen, always apply insect repellent after sunscreen.

Wear Long-Sleeved Shirts and Long Pants

To minimize the amount of exposed skin, wear long-sleeved shirts and long pants.

Treat Clothing and Gear with Permethrin

Use 0.5 percent permethrin to treat clothing and gear (such as boots, pants, socks, and tents) or buy permethrin-treated clothing and gear. Permethrin is an insecticide that kills or repels insects like mosquitoes and sand flies. Permethrin-treated clothing provides protection after multiple washings. Read product information to find out how long the protection will last. If treating items yourself, follow the product instructions. Do not use permethrin products directly on the skin. Watch the Centers for Disease Control and Prevention (CDC) video (www.cdc.gov/mosquitoes/mosquito-bites/how-to-use-permethrin.html) on how to use permethrin.

Keep Mosquitoes Out of Your Hotel Room or Lodging

- Choose a hotel or lodging with air conditioning or window and door screens.
- Use a mosquito net if you cannot stay in a place with air conditioning or window and door screens or if you are sleeping outside.

If mosquitoes bite you, avoid scratching the bites and apply over-the-counter (OTC) anti-itch or antihistamine cream to relieve itching.

Malaria is a serious disease that poses a significant risk to travelers in many parts of the world. Preventive measures, such as taking malaria medicine and using insect repellent, are essential. By following these guidelines, travelers can significantly reduce their risk of contracting malaria and ensure a safer journey.[1]

Section 23.6 | Schistosomiasis

Schistosomiasis, also known as "bilharzia" and "snail fever," is caused by helminth parasites of the genus *Schistosoma*.

TRANSMISSION OF SCHISTOSOMIASIS

Waterborne transmission occurs when larval cercariae, found in contaminated freshwater, penetrate the skin. Bathing, swimming, or wading in contaminated freshwater can result in infection. People of all ages are at risk. Human schistosomiasis is not acquired by contact with brackish or saltwater (oceans or seas). The distribution of schistosomiasis is very focal, determined by the presence of competent snail intermediate hosts, inadequate sanitation, and infected humans. Laboratory testing is required to determine if snails are infected with human schistosome species.

EPIDEMIOLOGY OF SCHISTOSOMIASIS

An estimated 85 percent of the world's cases of schistosomiasis are in Africa, where prevalence rates can exceed 50 percent in local populations. *Schistosoma mansoni* and *Schistosoma haematobium* are distributed throughout Africa. Only *S. haematobium* is found

---

[1] "Malaria," Centers for Disease Control and Prevention (CDC), September 13, 2022. Available online. URL: wwwnc.cdc.gov/travel/diseases/malaria. Accessed July 29, 2024.

in areas of the Middle East, and only *S. mansoni* in parts of Brazil, Suriname, and Venezuela. In the Caribbean, risk is very low, but *S. mansoni* is found in Guadeloupe, Martinique, and Saint Lucia, and previously in the Dominican Republic. *Schistosoma japonicum* is found in parts of China, Indonesia, and the Philippines. Although schistosomiasis had been eliminated in Europe for decades, transmission of *S. haematobium* was reported in Corsica in 2014. Two other species, *Schistosoma mekongi* (found in Cambodia and Laos) and *Schistosoma intercalatum* (found in parts of Central and West Africa), can infect humans but are rarely reported.

Many countries endemic for schistosomiasis have established control programs. Countries with widespread improvements in sanitation and water safety, especially those where successful control programs have been implemented, have likely eliminated this disease. No international guidelines currently exist for verifying elimination.

Adventure travelers, ecotourists, missionaries, Peace Corps volunteers, and soldiers are among travelers and expatriates at increased risk for infection. Outbreaks of schistosomiasis have occurred among adventure travelers on river trips in Africa. Most travel-associated cases of schistosomiasis are acquired in sub-Saharan Africa.

CLINICAL PRESENTATION

The incubation period for acute schistosomiasis is typically 14–84 days, and chronic asymptomatic infection can persist for years. Penetration of cercariae can cause a rash that develops within hours or up to a week after contaminated water exposure. Acute schistosomiasis (Katayama syndrome) is characterized by diarrhea, fever, headache, myalgia, and respiratory symptoms. Eosinophilia is often present; painful hepatomegaly or splenomegaly can also occur.

Clinical manifestations of chronic schistosomiasis result from host immune responses to schistosome eggs. *S. japonicum* and *S. mansoni* eggs most commonly lodge in the blood vessels of the liver or intestine, causing blood in the stool, constipation, and diarrhea. Chronic inflammation can lead to bowel wall ulceration, hyperplasia, polyposis, and, with heavy infections, to periportal liver fibrosis and splenomegaly. *S. haematobium* eggs typically lodge in the urinary tract, causing dysuria and hematuria. Calcifications in the bladder might appear late in the disease. *S. haematobium* infection can cause genital symptoms and has been associated with increased risk for bladder cancer. Rarely, central nervous system (CNS) manifestations develop, presenting as transverse myelitis.

DIAGNOSIS OF SCHISTOSOMIASIS

Diagnosis is made by microscopic identification of parasite eggs in stool (*S. japonicum* or *S. mansoni*) or urine (*S. haematobium*). Serologic tests are useful for diagnosing light infections, as egg shedding might not be consistent in travelers and in others who have not had schistosomiasis previously. Antibody tests do not distinguish between past and current infection but are useful for identifying infection in asymptomatic people who might have been exposed during travel and could benefit from treatment. Clinicians can obtain diagnostic assistance and confirmatory testing from the Centers for Disease Control and Prevention's (CDC) Division of Parasitic Diseases and Malaria (DPDM).

TREATMENT FOR SCHISTOSOMIASIS

Schistosomiasis is uncommon in the United States; clinicians unfamiliar with managing the condition should consult an infectious disease or tropical medicine specialist. Praziquantel is used to treat schistosomiasis and is most effective against adult forms of the parasite. Although a single course of treatment is usually curative, repeat treatment might be needed after two to four weeks to increase effectiveness in lightly infected patients.

PREVENTION OF SCHISTOSOMIASIS

No vaccine or drugs are available to prevent infection. Travelers can prevent schistosomiasis by avoiding bathing, swimming, wading, or other contact with freshwater in endemic countries. Untreated piped water from freshwater sources could contain cercariae; travelers should use fine-mesh filters, heat bathing water to 122 °F (50 °C) for five minutes, or allow water to stand for more than 24 hours before exposure.

Swimming in inadequately chlorinated pools is safe, even in endemic countries. Vigorous towel drying after accidental exposure to water has been suggested as a method of removing cercariae but should not generally be recommended as a preventive measure. Topical applications of insect repellents (e.g., N,N-diethyl-meta-toluamide, or DEET) can block penetrating cercariae but do not provide reliable coverage.

Schistosomiasis poses a significant health risk in many parts of the world, particularly in Africa. Travelers should be aware of the risk and take preventive measures to avoid infection.[1]

Section 23.7 | Sleeping Sickness (African Trypanosomiasis)

WHAT IS AFRICAN TRYPANOSOMIASIS?
African trypanosomiasis, also called "sleeping sickness," is a disease caused by a parasite. People can get this parasite when an infected tsetse fly bites them.

SYMPTOMS OF AFRICAN TRYPANOSOMIASIS
Symptoms include fatigue, high fever, headaches, and muscle aches. If the disease is not treated, it can cause death.

WHO IS AT RISK?
Tsetse flies are found in sub-Saharan Africa. Travelers who spend a lot of time outdoors or visit game parks in these areas can be bitten by them and become infected.

---

[1] "Schistosomiasis," Centers for Disease Control and Prevention (CDC), May 1, 2023. Available online. URL: wwwnc. cdc.gov/travel/yellowbook/2024/infections-diseases/schistosomiasis. Accessed July 29, 2024.

WHAT CAN TRAVELERS DO TO PREVENT AFRICAN TRYPANOSOMIASIS?

There is no vaccine or medicine that prevents African trypanosomiasis. Travelers can protect themselves by preventing tsetse fly bites.
Prevent tsetse fly bites by taking the following steps:

- **Cover exposed skin.** Wear long-sleeved shirts, long pants, and hats.
- **Choose appropriate clothing fabric.** It should be at least medium weight because the tsetse fly can bite through thin fabric.
- **Wear neutral-colored clothing.** The tsetse fly is attracted to bright colors, very dark colors, and metallic fabric, particularly blue and black.
- **Avoid bushes during the day.** The fly rests in bushes and will bite if disturbed.
- **Inspect vehicles for tsetse flies before entering.** The flies are attracted to the motion and dust from moving vehicles.
- **Use insect repellent.** Although there is limited evidence that insect repellent works against tsetse flies, it can prevent other diseases spread by bug bites.[1]

TREATMENT OPTIONS

Antitrypanosomal treatment is indicated for all persons diagnosed with human African trypanosomiasis (HAT). The choice of therapy depends on the parasite's infecting subspecies and the disease stage. The first-line drugs for both first- and second-stage disease are highly effective.

- Treatment during the first stage of *T. b. gambiense* infection:
  - **Pentamidine.** Used to treat first-stage *Trypanosoma brucei gambiense* infection in children under six years and under 20 kg without evidence of central

---

[1] "African Trypanosomiasis (African Sleeping Sickness)," Centers for Disease Control and Prevention (CDC), September 16, 2022. Available online. URL: wwwnc.cdc.gov/travel/diseases/african-sleeping-sickness-african-trypansosomiasis. Accessed July 29, 2024.

nervous system (CNS) disease. It is generally well-tolerated but may cause adverse reactions such as hypotension, hypoglycemia, injection site pain, diarrhea, nausea, and vomiting.

- **Fexinidazole**. It is now available as an oral alternative for treating first-stage *T. b. gambiense* infection in patients over six years of age and weighing over 20 kg.
- **Suramin**. Effective in treating the first stages of both *T. b. gambiense* and *T. b. rhodesiense* but recommended only for the first stage of *T. b. rhodesiense* due to the risk of severe adverse reactions in patients coinfected with onchocerciasis, which can occur in *T. b. gambiense*-endemic areas. Adverse reactions to suramin treatment in patients with *T. b. rhodesiense* trypanosomiasis are frequent but usually mild and reversible, including drug rash, nephrotoxicity, and peripheral neuropathy. In rare instances, suramin administration results in a hypersensitivity reaction; therefore, a small test dose is usually given before the full first dose.

- Treatment during the second stage of *T. b. gambiense* infection:
  - **Nifurtimox-eflornithine combination therapy (NECT) or fexinidazole (in patients over 6 years old weighing over 20 kg), depending on severity as measured by WBC in CSF and access to available regimens**. Limited data compares fexinidazole to NECT, but fexinidazole is preferred in low-resource settings given the ease of administration as an oral drug. The NECT combination regimen appears to be more effective and less toxic than eflornithine monotherapy. Adverse events with eflornithine include fever, pruritus, hypertension, nausea, vomiting, diarrhea, abdominal pain, headaches, myelosuppression, and more rarely, seizures. Eflornithine is not effective against *T. b. rhodesiense* and is not recommended for treating rhodesiense HAT.

- Treatment of *T. b. rhodesiense* infection:
  - **Suramin**. Currently used to treat first-stage *T. b. rhodesiense* infection.
  - **Melarsoprol**. An organoarsenic compound used to treat second-stage *T. b. rhodesiense*. Adverse reactions to melarsoprol can be severe and life-threatening. An encephalopathic reaction occurs in 5–10 percent of patients, with a case-fatality rate of approximately 50 percent when it occurs. Prednisone or prednisolone is often given to patients being treated with melarsoprol to reduce the risk of encephalopathy. Other adverse reactions observed with melarsoprol include gastrointestinal and skin reactions, pyrexia, and peripheral neuropathy. Intravenous injections of melarsoprol are painful and can cause phlebitis.

Consultation with a subject-matter expert at the Centers for Disease Control and Prevention (CDC) is advised to discuss treatment options for patients with *T. b. rhodesiense* and *T. b. gambiense* infections. There is no test or cure for HAT. After treatment, patients should be closely followed for 24 months and monitored for relapse. Recurrence of symptoms will require examination of body fluids, including CSF, to detect the presence of trypanosomes.[2]

---

[2] "Clinical Care of Human African Trypanosomiasis," Centers for Disease Control and Prevention (CDC), August 2, 2023. Available online. URL: www.cdc.gov/sleeping-sickness/hcp/clinical-care/index.html. Accessed July 29, 2024.

Chapter 24 | Other Health Risks

Chapter Contents

WHAT IS ALTITUDE ILLNESS?

If you plan to travel to an elevation higher than 8,000 feet above sea level, you may be at risk for altitude illness, which is caused by low oxygen levels in the air.

SYMPTOMS OF ALTITUDE ILLNESS

Acute mountain sickness (AMS) is the mildest form of altitude illness. Symptoms may include:

- headache
- tiredness
- lack of appetite
- nausea
- vomiting

Mild cases can be treated by easing symptoms, such as using pain relievers for a headache. Symptoms should go away on their own within a couple of days. People with altitude illness should not travel to higher elevations until they no longer have symptoms. A person whose symptoms get worse while resting should travel to a lower elevation to avoid becoming seriously ill or dying.

High-altitude cerebral edema (HACE) is a more serious form of AMS. Symptoms may include:

- extreme fatigue
- drowsiness
- confusion
- loss of coordination

High-altitude cerebral edema (HACE) is rare but can cause death. If it develops, the person must immediately move, or be moved, to a lower elevation.

High-altitude pulmonary edema (HAPE) is another serious form of altitude illness and can quickly become life-threatening. Symptoms include:

- shortness of breath
- weakness
- cough

A person with these symptoms must immediately move, or be moved, to a lower elevation and will likely need treatment with oxygen.

TIPS TO AVOID ALTITUDE ILLNESS

- **Ascend gradually**. Avoid traveling from a low elevation to an elevation higher than 9,000 feet (2,750 m) above sea level in one day. If possible, spend a few days at 8,000–9,000 feet before traveling to a higher elevation to give your body time to adjust to the lower oxygen levels.
- **Incremental increases**. Once you are above an elevation of 9,000 feet, increase where you sleep by no more than 1,600 feet per day. For every 3,300 feet you ascend, try to spend an extra day at that elevation without ascending further.
- **Avoid alcohol and heavy exercise**. Do not drink alcohol or engage in heavy exercise for at least the first 48 hours after you arrive at an elevation above 8,000 feet.
- **Pretravel acclimatization**. Traveling to elevations greater than 9,000 feet for two nights or more within 30 days before your trip can help avoid altitude illness on a longer trip at a high elevation.
- **Day trips for acclimatization**. Consider taking day trips to a higher elevation and then returning to a lower elevation to sleep.
- **Medications**. Medicines are available to prevent acute mountain sickness and shorten the time needed to get used to high elevations. Talk to your doctor about which is best for you given your medical history and trip plans. If your itinerary does not allow for gradual travel to a higher elevation, discuss with your doctor the medicine you can use to prevent or treat altitude illness. Many high-elevation destinations are remote, and access to medical care may be difficult.

Other Health Risks

PREEXISTING MEDICAL CONDITIONS
People with preexisting medical conditions should talk with a doctor before traveling to high elevations.

- **Heart or lung disease.** Consult a doctor familiar with high-altitude medicine before your trip.
- **Diabetes.** Be aware that managing diabetes may be more difficult at high elevations.
- **Pregnancy.** Pregnant women can make brief trips to high elevations but should talk with their doctor, as they may be advised not to sleep at elevations above 10,000 feet.
- **Severe conditions.** People with illnesses such as sickle cell anemia (SCA) and severe pulmonary hypertension should not travel to high elevations under any circumstances.

Altitude illness can pose significant risks for travelers ascending to high elevations. By following preventive measures, monitoring symptoms, and seeking medical advice when needed, travelers can enjoy high-altitude destinations safely.[1]

Section 24.2 | Blood Clots during Travel

UNDERSTANDING THE RISK OF BLOOD CLOTS
Traveling often involves sitting for extended periods, which can increase your chances of developing a deep vein thrombosis (DVT). DVT is a type of blood clot that forms in a large vein. If part of the clot breaks off, it can travel to the lungs and cause a pulmonary embolism (PE), a sudden blockage of arteries in the lung. Though these types of blood clots are rare, they are serious and can be life-threatening. Here are steps you can take to prevent blood clots during travel.

[1] "Travel to High Altitudes," Centers for Disease Control and Prevention (CDC), August 16, 2022. Available online. URL: wwwnc.cdc.gov/travel/page/travel-to-high-altitudes. Accessed July 30, 2024.

BLOOD CLOT RISK FACTORS

Sitting for a long time without getting up and walking around can cause blood to pool in the veins of your legs, increasing the risk of clots. Other conditions that elevate the risk include:

- a history of blood clots
- family history of blood clots
- known clotting disorder
- recent surgery, hospitalization, or injury
- use of estrogen-containing birth control or hormone replacement therapy (HRT)
- current or recent pregnancy
- older age
- obesity
- cancer or cancer treatments, such as chemotherapy
- serious medical conditions (e.g., congestive heart failure or inflammatory bowel disease (IBD))

PREVENT BLOOD CLOTS DURING TRAVEL

To reduce the risk of blood clots:

- **Stand up or walk occasionally.** When possible, select an aisle seat so you can move around every two to three hours.
- **Take breaks during car travel.** Include breaks in your schedule to stretch and walk around.
- **Exercise your calf muscles and stretch your legs while sitting.** Try these exercises:
  - Raise and lower your heels while keeping your toes on the floor.
  - Raise and lower your toes while keeping your heels on the floor.
  - Tighten and release your leg muscles.
- **Consult your doctor.** If you have additional risk factors for blood clots, discuss wearing compression stockings or taking medicine before departure. Taking aspirin to prevent blood clots when traveling is not recommended. If you take aspirin for other reasons, consult your doctor.

RECOGNIZE AND TREAT BLOOD CLOTS

Knowing the symptoms can help you recognize blood clots and seek timely medical care.

Deep Vein Thrombosis Symptoms
- swelling, pain, or tenderness in the affected area (usually the leg)
- unexplained pain or tenderness
- skin that is red and warm to the touch

Pulmonary Embolism Symptoms
- difficulty breathing
- faster than normal heartbeat
- chest pain that usually worsens with coughing or deep breathing
- coughing up blood
- lightheadedness or fainting

If you experience these symptoms, seek medical care immediately. Early detection and treatment can prevent severe complications or death.

DIAGNOSIS AND TREATMENT

To diagnose a DVT or PE, doctors may use various tests such as ultrasound, computed tomography (CT) scan, or magnetic resonance imaging (MRI). Treatment often involves medications or devices that dissolve, break up, remove, or capture the clot. Patients usually need to take medicine for several weeks or months to prevent new clots from forming and to allow the body to heal existing clots.

Blood clots during travel, though rare, can pose serious health risks. By understanding the risk factors and taking preventive measures, travelers can reduce their chances of developing DVT or PE.[1]

---

[1] "Prevent Blood Clots," Centers for Disease Control and Prevention (CDC), August 29, 2022. Available online. URL: wwwnc.cdc.gov/travel/page/dvt. Accessed July 30, 2024.

Section 24.3 | Food Poisoning from Marine Toxins

OVERVIEW OF MARINE TOXIN POISONING

Poisoning from ingesting marine toxins is an underrecognized hazard for travelers, particularly in the tropics and subtropics. Factors such as climate change, coral reef damage, expanding international trade and tourism, growing seafood consumption, and the spread of toxic algal blooms contribute to an increasing risk.

CIGUATERA FISH POISONING

Ciguatera fish poisoning occurs after eating reef fish contaminated with toxins such as ciguatoxin or maitotoxin. These potent toxins originate from *Gambierdiscus toxicus*, a small marine organism (dinoflagellate) that grows on coral reefs. Herbivorous fish ingest dinoflagellates, and the toxins produced are then modified and concentrated as they pass up the marine food chain to carnivorous fish and finally to humans. Ciguatoxins are concentrated in fish liver, intestines, roe, and heads.

Risk to Travelers

Approximately, 50,000 cases of ciguatera poisoning are reported worldwide annually, but the actual number is likely higher due to underreporting. Ciguatera poisoning is widespread in tropical and subtropical waters, particularly in the Pacific and Indian Oceans and the Caribbean Sea. The incidence and geographic distribution are increasing, with new risk areas including Madeira, the Canary Islands, parts of the Mediterranean, and the western Gulf of Mexico. Travelers may develop symptoms after returning home to nonendemic areas due to the increasing global trade in seafood products.

Large carnivorous reef fish (e.g., amberjack, barracuda, grouper, moray eel, sea bass, sturgeon) are most likely to cause ciguatera poisoning. Omnivorous and herbivorous fish (e.g., parrotfish, red snapper, surgeonfish) also pose a risk.

Clinical Presentation of Ciguatera Fish Poisoning

Ciguatera poisoning can cause cardiovascular, gastrointestinal (GI), neurologic, and neuropsychiatric illness. Symptoms typically develop within three to six hours after eating contaminated fish but can be delayed up to 30 hours. General symptoms include fatigue, malaise, and insomnia. Cardiovascular symptoms include bradycardia, heart block, or hypotension. Gastrointestinal symptoms include diarrhea, nausea, vomiting, and abdominal pain. Neurologic and neuropsychiatric symptoms include paresthesia, tooth pain, a burning or metallic taste, generalized itching, sweating, and blurred vision. Cold allodynia (abnormal sensation when touching cold water or objects) is a characteristic symptom, but acute sensitivity to both heat and cold can also be present. Neurologic symptoms usually last a few days to several weeks but can persist for months or even years.

The overall death rate from ciguatera poisoning is less than 0.1 percent but varies depending on the toxin dose and availability of medical care.

Treatment for Ciguatera Fish Poisoning

No specific antidote for ciguatoxin or maitotoxin poisoning exists. Symptomatic treatments include:

- amitriptyline for chronic paresthesias, depression, or pruritus
- fluoxetine for chronic fatigue
- gabapentin or pregabalin for neuropathic symptoms
- nifedipine or acetaminophen for headaches

Intravenous mannitol may reduce the severity and duration of neurologic symptoms if given within 48 hours of symptom onset. After recovery, patients should avoid alcohol, caffeine, fish, and nuts for at least six months to prevent symptom relapse.

Prevention of Ciguatera Fish Poisoning

To prevent ciguatera fish poisoning, travelers should avoid or limit the consumption of reef fish, especially fish weighing more than

5 pounds. They should also avoid high-risk fish (e.g., barracuda, and moray eel) and the parts of fish that concentrate ciguatera toxin (e.g., head, intestines, liver, and roe).

SCOMBROID POISONING

Scombroid poisoning occurs after consuming fish with high levels of histamine, which result from improper storage. Fish typically associated with scombroid include amberjack, anchovies, blue-fish, herring, mackerel, mahi mahi, marlin, sardines, and tuna. Proper storage can mitigate the process of histidine conversion to histamine.

Clinical Presentation of Scombroid Poisoning

Symptoms of scombroid poisoning resemble an acute aller-gic reaction and appear 10–60 minutes after eating contami-nated fish. Signs include abdominal cramps, diarrhea, blurred vision, facial flushing, severe headaches, itching, and palpita-tions. Symptoms typically resolve within 12–48 hours without long-term sequelae.

Treatment and Prevention of Scombroid Poisoning

Treatment usually involves antihistamines. Prevention includes proper refrigeration or icing of fish to prevent histamine production.

SHELLFISH POISONING

Shellfish poisoning occurs when shellfish harbor toxins from small marine organisms. Contaminated shellfish can be found in tem-perate and tropical waters, typically during or after harmful algal blooms (HABs).

Types of Shellfish Poisoning

- **Amnesic shellfish poisoning (ASP).** Caused by domoic acid, symptoms include GI issues and cognitive impairment.
- **Diarrheic shellfish poisoning (DSP).** Caused by okadaic acid, symptoms include abdominal pain and diarrhea.

- **Neurotoxic shellfish poisoning (NSP).** Caused by brevetoxins, symptoms include gastroenteritis and neurologic effects.
- **Paralytic shellfish poisoning (PSP).** The most severe, caused by saxitoxins, symptoms include numbness, tingling, and respiratory failure.

Treatment and Prevention of Shellfish Poisoning

Treatment is symptomatic and supportive. Severe cases of PSP may require mechanical ventilation. Prevention involves avoiding shellfish from areas affected by algal blooms and ensuring proper preparation methods.

Marine toxin poisoning poses significant health risks, especially in tropical and subtropical regions. Awareness, preventive measures, and prompt medical attention are essential for travelers to manage and mitigate these risks effectively.[1]

Section 24.4 | Jet Lag

Jet lag results from a mismatch between a person's circadian (24-hour) rhythms and the time of day in a new time zone. When establishing the risk of jet lag, first determine how many time zones a traveler will cross and what the discrepancy will be between the time of day at home and at the destination upon arrival. During the first few days after a flight to a new time zone, a person's circadian rhythms are still anchored to the time of day at their initial departure location. These rhythms then gradually adjust to the new time zone.

For travelers crossing three or fewer time zones, especially on long-haul flights, symptoms (e.g., tiredness) are likely due to fatigue

---

[1] "Food Poisoning from Marine Toxins," Centers for Disease Control and Prevention (CDC), May 1, 2023. Available online. URL: wwwnc.cdc.gov/travel/yellowbook/2024/environmental-hazards-risks/food-poisoning-from-marine-toxins. Accessed July 30, 2024.

rather than jet lag, and these symptoms should abate one to three days postflight.

Many people flying across more than three time zones for a vacation accept the risk of jet lag as a transient and mild inconvenience. However, people traveling on business or competing in athletic events might seek advice on prophylactic measures and treatments. If a traveler spends two or fewer days in the new time zone, they might prefer to anchor their sleep-wake schedule to the time of day at home as much as possible. Consider recommending short-acting hypnotics or alertness-enhancing drugs (e.g., caffeine) for such travelers to minimize the total burden of jet lag during short round trips.

CLINICAL PRESENTATION

Jet lag symptoms can be difficult to define because of individual variations and because the same person can experience different symptoms after each flight. Jet-lagged travelers typically experience one or more of the following symptoms after flying across more than three time zones: gastrointestinal (GI) disturbances, decreased interest in or enjoyment of meals, negative feelings (e.g., anxiety, depression, fatigue, headache, inability to concentrate, irritability), poor performance of physical and mental tasks during the new daytime, and classically, poor sleep. This includes difficulty initiating sleep at the usual time of night (after eastward flights), early awakening (after westward flights), and fractionated sleep (after flights in either direction).

Symptoms are difficult to distinguish from general fatigue resulting from international travel and other travel factors (e.g., hypoxia in the aircraft cabin). Validated multi-symptom measurement tools (e.g., Liverpool Jet Lag Index) can help differentiate jet lag from fatigue. When travelers cross only one or two time zones, symptoms and treatment for jet lag are not readily distinguishable from those for general travel fatigue.

In addition to jet lag symptoms, crossing multiple time zones can affect the timing of regular medication used for chronic conditions and illnesses, particularly for patients taking medications with short half-lives that require more than one dose each day. When evaluating travelers who take long-term medications, consider the destination and travel time and recommend strategies to keep them on their dosing schedule.

PREVENTION AND TREATMENT

Travelers use various approaches before, during, and after flying to reduce jet lag symptoms. In one survey, 460 long-haul travelers indicated that seat selection and booking a direct flight were primary strategies to reduce jet lag. Nearly all study participants used one or more behavioral strategies during their flight, including consuming or avoiding alcohol and caffeine (81%), altering food intake (68%), using light exposure (53%), periodic walking down the aisle of the plane (35%), and taking medication (15%), including melatonin (8%). Only one respondent used a jet lag application on a mobile device. Fewer people used all these strategies before take-off and after arrival.

After arrival, light and social contacts influence the timing of internal circadian rhythms. A traveler staying in the time zone for more than two days should quickly try to adjust to the local sleep-wake schedule as much as possible.

Diet and Physical Activity

Most dietary interventions or functional foods have not been proven to reduce jet lag symptoms in randomized controlled trials (RCTs) and real flight conditions. Most trials are conducted in simulated flight conditions and have a high risk of bias. This includes studies examining the effectiveness of *Centella asiatica*, elderberry, echinacea, pinokinase, and diets containing various levels of fiber, fluids, or macronutrients. In one study, long-haul flight crew who adopted more regular mealtimes showed a small improvement in their general subjective rating of jet lag, but not the separate symptoms of alertness or jet lag, on their days off work.

Because GI disturbance is a common jet lag symptom, travelers might better tolerate smaller meals than larger ones before and during the flight; this strategy has not been investigated in a formal trial. Travelers might find caffeine and physical activity can help ameliorate daytime sleepiness at the destination, but little evidence exists to indicate that these interventions reduce overall feelings of jet lag. Any purported treatments based on acupressure, aromatherapy, or homeopathy lack a scientific basis.

Hypnotic Medications

Prescription medications (e.g., temazepam, zolpidem, zopiclone) can reduce sleep loss during and after travel but do not necessarily help resynchronize circadian rhythms or improve overall jet lag symptoms. If indicated, prescribe the lowest effective dose of a short- to medium-acting compound for the initial few days of travel, bearing in mind these drugs have adverse effects. In 2019, the U.S. Food and Drug Administration (FDA) issued a warning about rare but serious adverse events (i.e., injuries caused by sleepwalking) occurring after patients took some sleep medications; these events were more commonly reported with eszopiclone, zaleplon, and zolpidem.

Caution travelers about taking hypnotics during a flight, as the resulting immobility could increase the risk of deep vein thrombosis (DVT). Travelers should not use alcohol as a sleep aid because it disrupts sleep and can provoke obstructive sleep apnea (OSA).

Light

Exposure to bright light can advance or delay human circadian rhythms depending on when it is received in relation to a person's body clock time. Consequently, some researchers have proposed schedules for good and bad times for light exposure after arrival in a new time zone.

The best circadian time for light exposure might be dark after crossing multiple time zones, raising the question whether a light box is helpful. One small RCT on supplementary bright light for reducing jet lag did not find clinically relevant effects of supplementary light on jet lag symptoms after a flight across five time zones going west.

Melatonin and Melatonin-Receptor Analogs

Melatonin, probably the most well-known treatment for jet lag, is secreted at night by the pineal gland. When taken during the rising phase of body temperature (usually the morning), melatonin delays circadian rhythms and advances rhythms when ingested during the falling phase (usually the evening). These effects are opposite to those of bright light.

Most product instructions advise travelers to take melatonin before nocturnal sleep in the new time zone, irrespective of the number of time zones crossed or the direction of travel. Studies published in the mid-1980s indicated a substantial benefit of taking melatonin just before sleep to reduce overall feelings of jet lag after flights. Subsequent larger studies did not replicate these earlier findings, and more research on melatonin's use in jet lag is needed.

Melatonin is a very popular sleep aid for jet lag in the United States, and no serious side effects have been linked to its use, although long-term studies have not been conducted. The American Academy of Sleep Medicine (AASM) and the U.S. National Center for Complementary and Integrative Health (NCCIH) suggest that melatonin could be used to reduce symptoms of jet lag, although they caution that melatonin might not be safe when combined with some other medications. In addition, melatonin is considered a dietary supplement in the United States and is not regulated by the FDA. Therefore, the advertised melatonin concentration has not been confirmed for most products on the market, and the presence of contaminants cannot be ruled out.

A UK Drug and Therapeutics Bulletin (DTB) stated that melatonin might increase the frequency of seizures in people with epilepsy. Additionally, because it can potentially induce pro-inflammatory cytokine production, melatonin should not be taken by those with autoimmune diseases. Due to these potential problems and the limited evidence from RCTs for any benefits, melatonin is not recommended in the United Kingdom.

Ramelteon, a melatonin-receptor agonist, is an FDA-approved treatment for insomnia. One milligram taken just before bedtime can decrease sleep onset latency after eastward travel across five time zones. Higher doses do not seem to lead to further improvements, and the effect of this medication on other symptoms of jet lag and the timing of circadian rhythms is unclear. In a well-designed multicenter trial involving simulated jet lag conditions, tasimelteon (a dual melatonin-receptor agonist) improved jet lag symptoms, including vnighttime insomnia and daytime functioning.

Real-world evidence is needed to support or refute its use in ameliorating jet lag.

Mobile Applications

Several mobile device applications can provide tailored advice to manage jet lag symptoms, depending on how many time zones the traveler has crossed. Timeshifter advises when to use caffeine, light, melatonin, and sleep. Another app offering tailored advice was tested over several months of frequent flying. Participants reported reduced fatigue compared with the comparator group and improved aspects of health-related behavior (e.g., physical activity, snacking, and sleep quality) but not other measures of sleep (e.g., duration, latency, use of sleep-related medication). Although this and other apps are based on information from published laboratory-based experiments, they lack RCTs on their effectiveness for reducing jet lag symptoms after actual long-haul flights.

Combination Treatments

Multiple therapies to decrease jet lag symptoms can be combined into treatment packages. Marginal gains from multiple treatments could aggregate. In one small trial, a treatment package involving light exposure and sleep hygiene advice improved sleep quality and physical performance after an eastward flight across eight time zones. The American Sleep Association offers general sleep hygiene advice.

In general, no cure is available for jet lag. Instead, counseling should focus on factors known from laboratory simulations to alter circadian timing. Until more RCTs of treatments prescribed before, during, or after transmeridian flights are published, robust, evidence-based advice should be provided.[1]

---

[1] "Jet Lag," Centers for Disease Control and Prevention (CDC), May 1, 2023. Available online. URL: wwwnc.cdc.gov/travel/yellowbook/2024/air-land-sea/jet-lag. Accessed July 30, 2024.

Section 24.5 | Motion Sickness

Motion sickness describes the physiological responses to travel by air, car, sea, train, and virtual reality immersion. Given sufficient stimulus, all people with functional vestibular systems can develop motion sickness. However, individuals vary in their susceptibility.

RISK FOR TRAVELERS

Risk factors for motion sickness include age, sex, preexisting medical conditions, and concurrent medications. Children aged 2–12 years are especially susceptible, but infants and toddlers are generally immune. Adults over 50 years are less susceptible to motion sickness. Pregnancy, menstruation, and taking hormone replacement therapy (HRT) or oral contraceptives have also been identified as potential risk factors. People with a history of migraines, vertigo, and vestibular disorders are more prone to motion sickness. Some prescriptions can worsen motion sickness-associated nausea.

CLINICAL PRESENTATION

Motion sickness typically occurs after a triggering motion or event. People with motion sickness commonly experience dizziness, headache, nausea, vomiting or retching, and sweating. A complete list of motion sickness-associated signs and symptoms includes the following:

- **Anorexia.** Loss of appetite or reduced desire to eat.
- **Apathy.** Lack of interest or concern.
- **Cold sweats.** Sweating accompanied by a cold, clammy feeling.
- **Drowsiness.** A state of being tired and ready to fall asleep.
- **Generalized discomfort.** A general sense of unease or physical discomfort.
- **Headache.** Pain in the head or face area.
- **Hyperventilation.** Rapid or deep breathing.

- **Increased sensitivity to odors**. Heightened awareness of smells.
- **Nausea**. An uneasy sensation often leading to vomiting.
- **Excessive salivation**. Increased production of saliva.
- **Sweating**. Increased perspiration.
- **Vomiting or retching**. Expulsion of stomach contents or dry heaving.
- **Warm sensation**. Feeling warm without an increase in body temperature.

NEUROPHYSIOLOGY

When sensory input does not align with expected patterns (neural mismatch), patients may experience dizziness and nausea. The sensory conflict theory, the most widely accepted explanation for motion sickness, proposes that the condition results from a conflict between the visual, vestibular, and somatosensory systems. This involves complex neurophysiological signaling between multiple nuclear regions, neurotransmitters, and receptors. Medications used to prevent and treat motion sickness are thought to work by suppressing the signals contributing to neural mismatch.

NONPHARMACOLOGIC PREVENTION AND INTERVENTIONS

Travelers can use nonpharmacologic interventions to prevent or treat motion sickness. Awareness and avoidance of situations that tend to trigger symptoms are primary defenses against motion sickness:

- **Be aware**. Try to avoid situations that tend to trigger your symptoms.
- **Optimize your position**. Reduce motion or motion perception by driving a vehicle instead of riding in it, sitting in the front seat of a car or bus, sitting over the wing of an aircraft, holding your head firmly against the back of the seat, or choosing a window seat on flights and trains.

- **Reduce sensory input**. Lie face down, shut your eyes, try sleeping, or look at the horizon.
- **Maintain hydration**. Drink water, eat small meals frequently, and limit alcoholic and caffeinated beverages.
- **Get plenty of sleep or rest**. Being sleep-deprived can worsen motion sickness symptoms.
- **Avoid smoking**. Quitting, even short-term, reduces susceptibility to motion sickness.
- **Try using distractions**. Controlled breathing, listening to music, or using aromatherapy scents, such as mint, lavender, or ginger. Flavored lozenges might also help.

Some people recommend using acupressure or magnets to prevent or treat nausea, although scientific data are lacking on their effectiveness for preventing motion sickness.

Gradually exposing oneself to continuous or repeated motion sickness triggers may help reduce symptoms over time.

TREATMENT FOR MOTION SICKNESS

Medications used to treat motion sickness can vary in effectiveness and side effects. Travelers should take a trial dose of medication at home before departure to determine what works best for them. The most frequently used antihistamines for treating motion sickness include cyclizine, dimenhydrinate, meclizine, and promethazine (oral and suppository). Nonsedating antihistamines appear to be less effective. Other commonly used medications include anticholinergics (e.g., scopolamine), benzodiazepines, dopamine receptor antagonists (e.g., metoclopramide, prochlorperazine), and sympathomimetics (often used in combination with antihistamines).

Complementary approaches with anecdotal evidence of effectiveness for preventing or treating motion sickness, such as acupressure and magnets, ginger, homeopathic remedies, and pyridoxine (vitamin B_6), might be effective for individual travelers but cannot generally be recommended. Clinical trials have shown that ondansetron, a commonly used antiemetic, is ineffective in preventing nausea associated with motion sickness.

Understanding risk factors and effective interventions can help mitigate motion sickness symptoms, making travel more comfortable.[1]

Section 24.6 | Sun Protection and Safety for Travelers

When you are outdoors, you may be exposed to the sun's harmful ultraviolet (UV) rays. Prolonged UV exposure can lead to both short-term issues such as sunburns and long-term problems such as sun damage, premature aging, and skin cancer. Your risk for UV exposure may be higher depending on your activities and travel destinations.

PROTECT YOURSELF FROM THE SUN

You are at the greatest risk for UV exposure when traveling near the equator, during the summer months, at high elevations, or between 10 a.m. and 4 p.m. UV rays can also penetrate clouds and reflect off surfaces like snow, sand, and water, increasing exposure even on cloudy days and in winter. Therefore, protecting yourself from the sun during any outdoor activities is crucial.

USE SUNSCREEN

Sunscreen protects you from sun exposure by reflecting or absorbing UV rays. Follow these tips when selecting and applying sunscreen:

- Use sun protection factor (SPF) 15 or higher.
- Ensure your sunscreen "blocks ultraviolet A (UVA) and ultraviolet B (UVB)" or has "broad spectrum" on the label.

---

[1] "Motion Sickness," Centers for Disease Control and Prevention (CDC), May 1, 2023. Available online. URL: wwwnc.cdc.gov/travel/yellowbook/2024/air-land-sea/motion-sickness. Accessed July 30, 2024.

- Apply sunscreen to create a thick layer on the skin at least 20 minutes before sun exposure.
- Apply sunscreen to all exposed skin, including ears, scalp, lips, neck, tops of feet, and backs of hands.
- Reapply at least every two hours.
- Reapply each time you exit water or sweat heavily.
- Apply sunscreen first if using insect repellent and insect repellent second. Follow the product label instructions to determine how often to reapply both.
- Dispose of sunscreen containers after one to two years.

WEAR PROTECTIVE CLOTHING
- Wear clothing to cover as much skin as possible.
- Wear a hat with a wide brim to shade the face, head, ears, and neck.
- Wear sunglasses that block both UVA and UVB rays.

TAKE ADDITIONAL STEPS
- Stay in the shade, especially during midday hours (10 a.m. to 4 p.m.).
- Drink plenty of nonalcoholic fluids.
- Avoid indoor tanning facilities. Getting a "base tan" before your vacation damages your skin and does not protect you from sun exposure on your trip.

HOW TO TREAT A SUNBURN
- Take aspirin, acetaminophen, or ibuprofen to relieve pain, headache, and fever.
- Drink plenty of water.
- Soothe burns with cool baths or by gently applying cool, wet cloths.
- Use a topical moisturizing cream or aloe to provide additional relief.
- Avoid further sun exposure until the burn has healed.
- If your skin blisters, lightly bandage or cover the area with gauze to prevent infection. Do not break blisters, as this

can slow healing and increase the risk of infection. Apply antiseptic ointment if blisters break.

- Seek medical attention if you have a severe sunburn, especially if it covers more than 15 percent of your body, causes dehydration, involves a high fever, or results in extreme pain lasting more than 48 hours.[1]

Section 24.7 | Toxic Exposures and Poisonous Substances for Travelers

Travelers outside the United States may encounter unfamiliar substances that can harm their health. Local and regional poison centers can provide information and medical guidance in cases of suspected poisoning or other toxic exposures. These centers employ specialists knowledgeable about indigenous poisonous fauna and flora and their available treatments. The World Health Organization (WHO) offers a comprehensive list of poison centers and important contact information for many countries. Operating hours and availability to the public may vary.

TOXIC EXPOSURES
Carbon Monoxide
Carbon monoxide (CO) is an odorless, colorless, and nonirritating gas produced during the combustion of carbon-based fuels (e.g., charcoal, gasoline, and propane). Symptoms associated with CO inhalation include dizziness, headache, nausea, vomiting, shortness of breath, loss of consciousness, and death. CO poisoning can have long-term neurologic effects even after removal from exposure. Children and small pets often experience symptoms sooner than adults due to their higher respiratory rates. Deaths due to CO

---

[1] "Sun Exposure," Centers for Disease Control and Prevention (CDC), August 16, 2022. Available online. URL: wwwnc.cdc.gov/travel/page/sun-exposure. Accessed July 30, 2024.

poisoning have been reported among international travelers staying in hotels and rented apartments.

Chemical Irritants

In response to popular protests or civil unrest, law enforcement and military forces sometimes deploy chemical irritants, also known as "crowd control agents," "lacrimators," or "tear gas." These substances are intended to cause tearing of the eyes and pain without permanent injury, although cases of lasting disability and death have been reported. Chemical irritants can cause breathing problems (e.g., chest tightness, choking sensation, coughing, and shortness of breath). International travelers should be aware of areas where popular protests or other mass gatherings are planned or commonly occur. U.S. citizens can enroll in the U.S. Department of State's (DOS) free Smart Traveler Enrollment Program (STEP) to receive information from the local U.S. Embassy or Consulate about safety and security concerns.

Herbicides, Pesticides, and Rodenticides

Herbicides, pesticides, and rodenticides help reduce pests and the diseases they carry. All pesticides available for use in the United States are registered with the Environmental Protection Agency (EPA) and evaluated for safety. However, other countries may use pesticides deemed illegal, unsafe, or improperly labeled in the United States. Travelers visiting or working in rural areas may encounter agricultural insecticides or herbicides applied over large areas, often without proper personal protective equipment or other measures to prevent exposure. In urban areas, highly toxic substances such as organophosphates, metal phosphides, and arsenic-containing compounds may be used to control pests. Several cases of deaths among tourists have been reported, where pesticides used to fumigate hotel rooms were suspected to have played a role.

FOOD AND BEVERAGE POISONING
Alcohol

Risks associated with consuming alcohol outside the United States include the possibility of drinking contaminated or adulterated products. This is particularly true in countries where regulations and standards for distilling and distributing alcohol are less strict. Homemade alcoholic beverages (moonshine), often produced under unsafe and unsanitary conditions, might contain contaminants, impurities, or unusually high levels of ethanol, increasing the risk of alcohol poisoning.

Botulism

Botulism is a potentially deadly disease caused by a toxin produced by the bacterium *Clostridium botulinum*. Symptoms initially include blurred vision, difficulty speaking, and weakness but can progress to paralysis. The illness may manifest and be transmitted in multiple ways, including foodborne botulism, wound botulism, and infant botulism.

Most pertinent to international travel is foodborne botulism, caused by eating food contaminated with the botulinum toxin. Although the United States has food safety guidelines for canned and preserved foods, other countries may not. Preserved foods, including smoked fishes and other cured meats, can pose a risk if not stored at proper temperatures. Pickled or preserved foods also pose a risk if they do not contain the proper amounts of salt or acidity. Medical tourists are at risk of iatrogenic botulism, which can result when too much botulinum toxin is injected to treat conditions such as chronic pain, excessive sweating, migraine headaches, muscle spasticity, obesity, or wrinkles.

Foraging

Foraging for wild edible plants and mushrooms can be a fun and interesting way to learn about nature and find food in international destinations, but it can also be dangerous. Edible plants and fungi in one country may have deadly look-alikes in another. Travelers who wish to forage should use a region-specific field or foraging guides and educate themselves on possible dangerous look-alikes. There are sometimes legal issues surrounding foraging. For example, it can be illegal to forage for plants or mushrooms without permission from landowners, and the act of harvesting itself can be illegal for certain plants and mushrooms.

ZOONOTIC EXPOSURES (ENVENOMATIONS)

Animals use venom to defend themselves or subdue prey, delivering toxic substances by biting or stinging. Venom often consists of complex mixtures of molecules that can affect a victim's blood, muscle tissue, nervous system, or other organs.

Cnidarians

Recreational activities in the ocean (e.g., scuba diving, snorkeling, and swimming) can lead to encounters with marine animals that can sting or bite. Cnidarians include corals, hydroids (e.g., fire coral, Portuguese man o' war), jellyfish, and sea anemones. These organisms have highly developed stinging structures (nematocysts) on their tentacles that can penetrate the skin and cause pain and irritation. Many cnidarian stings cause painful and itching rashes but are not typically associated with severe illness. Seabather's eruption is a rash caused by cnidarian larvae that become trapped (e.g., under a bathing suit). Fire coral is a frequent cause of stings among divers in the Caribbean. Jellyfish are encountered at beaches worldwide.

Fish

Certain types of fish (e.g., lionfish, stingrays, and stonefish) possess sharp venomous spines that can injure humans. Hot-water immersion may limit the effects of venom from spiny fish. Many injured people require medical treatment for pain control, wound care, and removal of embedded foreign material.

Sea Urchins and Sea Stars

Sea urchins can cause severe puncture wounds, especially when stepped on. The venom on their spines can cause intense burning pain, redness, and swelling of the injured areas. Rare reports of illness following sea urchin envenomation have been reported, although the clinical effects are not well documented. Sea urchin spines can be brittle and difficult to remove; retained spines can cause severe inflammation, infection, and scar tissue formation. Hot-water immersion can help limit the effects of sea urchin and starfish venoms. Medical attention may be needed to remove spines because they are often brittle and crumble easily. Travelers not up to date with tetanus vaccines may require a booster and, in some cases, antibiotics to prevent bacterial infections associated with puncture wounds in the marine environment.

Scorpions

Scorpions can be found on every continent except Antarctica but are most commonly seen in subtropical and tropical areas. Scorpion stings often cause intense pain and redness, but venom from some species can cause severe illness, affecting the heart, nervous system, and other organs. Manifestations include agitation, arrhythmias, bleeding and other coagulation disorders, pancreatitis, uncontrollable muscle spasms, shock, and even death. While most scorpion stings are not serious, medical attention may be needed for pain management and wound care, including preventive tetanus vaccine. Young children may be more likely to develop neurologic symptoms and need urgent treatment. People with severe symptoms of envenomation may require hospitalization and antivenoms, if available. Preventive measures to avoid scorpion stings include shaking out clothing and shoes before putting them on and wearing long-sleeved shirts and long pants when walking in areas with scorpions.

Snakes

Many snake species possess venom used to immobilize or kill prey. In humans, snakebites can cause serious injury, disability, or even death. In 2019, an estimated 63,400 deaths worldwide were attributed to snakebites. Access to prompt medical treatment is the most important measure to limit the extent of injury and illness following a snakebite, and delayed access to care can be life-threatening. Treatment often requires antivenom, which could be difficult to obtain in remote areas. When traveling in areas with venomous snakes, it is prudent to obtain information about the location of the closest medical facility, availability of antivenom, and resources for transportation to a larger hospital if needed.

Spiders

Most encounters with spiders are harmless and do not result in injury or illness. Some spiders, however, capture and immobilize prey using venom, potentially harming humans. Spiders are shy and typically do not attack humans without provocation but may bite in self-defense if disturbed. Reports of spider bites are often unreliable because people commonly mistake skin wounds and infections for spider bites, even if no spider was seen.

Travelers may encounter a wide range of toxic exposures and poisonous substances while abroad. Awareness and precautionary measures, such as avoiding unfamiliar foods, using protective clothing, and staying informed about local hazards, are essential for minimizing risks. In case of exposure, knowing the location of the nearest medical facilities and poison centers can be life-saving.[1]

[1] "Poisonings, Envenomations, and Toxic Exposures," Centers for Disease Control and Prevention (CDC), May 22, 2023. Available online. URL: wwwnc.cdc.gov/travel/yellowbook/2024/environmental-hazards-risks/poisonings-envenomations-and-toxic-exposures. Accessed July 30, 2024.

Part 4 | **Modes of Travel and Shelters**

Chapter 25 | Travel Modes and Safety

Section 25.1 | Road Safety

Roads, signs, laws, and driving norms often differ abroad. Prioritize your safety by ensuring you have a valid license and insurance. Always remember to buckle up, no matter where you are.

For more information, check the foreign embassy or consulate website (www.usembassy.gov). Government tourism offices or car rental companies may also provide helpful resources.

Keep these considerations in mind when planning your trip:

- **Potential hazards and dangerous road conditions**. Be aware of any known issues.
- **Local roads or areas to avoid**. Some regions may be unsafe for travel.
- **Need for spare tires, fuel, and a map**. Prepare for emergencies.
- **Local laws and driving culture**. Understand the rules and customs.
- **Local emergency numbers**. Have them readily available.
- **Vehicle safety considerations, including seat belts**. Ensure your vehicle is equipped.
- **Documents to carry, including any special road permits**. Verify necessary paperwork.
- **Insurance and driver's license**. Check requirements and validity.

INTERNATIONAL DRIVING PERMITS

It is illegal to drive without a valid license and insurance in most countries. While not all countries accept a U.S. driver's license, most recognize an international driving permit (IDP). You can obtain an IDP from the American Automobile Association (AAA) before you leave. IDPs have limited validity and usually require you to carry your U.S. license as well.

AUTO INSURANCE POLICIES

Generally, U.S. auto insurance policies do not cover you abroad, although some may provide coverage in Canada and Mexico.

Confirm with your insurance company before traveling. Even if your policy is valid in a country, it may not meet local insurance minimums. Make sure your policy complies with these minimums. While rental companies overseas may offer car insurance, it might be for a minimal amount. Consider purchasing additional coverage to match what you have at home.[1]

Plan long trips carefully, and monitor the radio or television for up-to-date weather forecasts and road conditions. Drive only if absolutely necessary in bad weather.

PREPARE YOUR CAR FOR EMERGENCIES

Have a mechanic check the following on your car:

- **Antifreeze levels**. Prevents the engine from freezing.
- **Battery and ignition system**. Ensure reliable starts.
- **Brakes**. Essential for safe stopping.
- **Exhaust system**. Check for leaks that could allow carbon monoxide into the car.
- **Fuel and air filters**. Replace as needed for efficiency.
- **Heater and defroster**. Ensure proper function for visibility and comfort.
- **Lights and flashing hazard lights**. Verify all lights are working.
- **Oil**. Change as needed.
- **Thermostat**. Ensure it regulates engine temperature properly.
- **Windshield wiper equipment and washer fluid level**. For clear visibility.

EMERGENCY KIT FOR THE CAR

In case you are stranded, keep an emergency supply kit in your car with these extras:

- **Jumper cables**. To restart your vehicle if the battery dies.
- **Flares or reflective triangle**. To signal for help and warn other drivers.

---

[1] Bureau of Consular Affairs, "Driving and Road Safety Abroad," U.S. Department of State (DOS), March 5, 2024. Available online. URL: https://travel.state.gov/content/travel/en/international-travel/before-you-go/driving-and-road-safety.html. Accessed July 30, 2024.

- **Ice scraper**. For clearing ice from windows.
- **Car cell phone charger**. To keep your phone charged in emergencies.
- **Blanket**. For warmth if stranded in cold weather.
- **Map**. For navigation without the Global Positioning System (GPS).
- **Cat litter or sand**. For better tire traction in snow or ice.

CAR SAFETY TIPS

- **Keep your gas tank full**. This is crucial in case of evacuation or power outages and prevents the fuel line from freezing.
- **Install good winter tires**. Ensure they have enough tread or use chains or studs if required in your area.
- **Avoid driving through flooded areas**. As little as six inches of water can cause a vehicle to lose control or stall, and a foot of water can float many cars.
- **Be cautious in areas where floodwaters have receded**. Roads may be weakened and could collapse under a vehicle's weight.
- **If a power line falls on your car, stay inside**. You risk electrical shock until a trained person removes the wire.
- **Pull over if the car becomes hard to control**. Stop and set the parking brake.
- **Avoid hazards**. Avoid overpasses, bridges, power lines, signs, and other dangers during emergencies.[2]

RESEARCH YOUR DESTINATION

Customs and norms in other countries can differ significantly from those in the United States. Check the country information pages (https://travel.state.gov/content/travel/en/international-travel/International-Travel-Country-Information-Pages.html) for specific information on visa requirements, safety and security

---

[2] Ready.gov, "Car Safety," U.S. Department of Homeland Security (DHS), April 15, 2024. Available online. URL: www.ready.gov/car. Accessed July 30, 2024.

conditions, crime, health considerations, local laws, areas to avoid, and more. Enroll in the Smart Traveler Enrollment Program (STEP; https://step.state.gov/step) to receive information about health and safety in your destination country. Enrolling in STEP also allows the U.S. Embassy or Consulate to contact you in case of an emergency.

BE AWARE OF LOCAL CUSTOMS AND NORMS

Some countries have rules or norms different from those in the United States. For example, tight-fitting clothes, sleeveless shirts, and shorts may be unacceptable in certain regions. Pack accordingly and review country information pages for guidance.

FREEDOM OF SPEECH

While some countries have laws protecting free speech and peaceful assembly similar to the United States, others may have more restrictive laws. Discussing sensitive subjects openly or posting on social media can lead to fines or arrest in some countries. Consult the State Department's Human Rights reports (www.state.gov/reports-bureau-of-democracy-human-rights-and-labor/country-reports-on-human-rights-practices) for specific country information.

PROHIBITED ITEMS

Check the customs and import restrictions page for items not allowed into or out of your destination country. Restrictions may apply to items such as over-the-counter (OTC) medications, drugs, alcohol, contraceptives, religious items, and literature. Items permitted in the United States might be restricted elsewhere.

PUBLIC TRANSPORT

Public transportation safety varies by country. In many places, informal taxis or minibuses can be dangerous, especially for solo travelers. Reliable sources, such as local authorities or tourism officials, can provide information on safe transport options.

Consider these transport tips:

- **Arrange transport to and from the airport before arrival**. Use licensed and reputable companies.
- **Do not hitchhike**. It can be unsafe.
- **Research taxi and ride-share companies**. Ensure they are licensed and reputable.
- **Use app-based transportation companies**. These companies offer ride records, unlike street-hail taxis. Some apps allow real-time ride-sharing with a trusted contact.
- **Avoid crowded public transportation**. It can be a hotspot for pickpockets.

TRAVEL ACCOMMODATIONS

Review the lodging safety (https://travel.state.gov/content/travel/en/international-travel/before-you-go/lodging-safety.html) and follow these tips:

- **Research accommodations carefully**. Read reviews for safety concerns and have backup options.
- **Arrange your accommodation before you travel**. You are more vulnerable in unfamiliar surroundings upon arrival.
- **Do not share your accommodation details with strangers**. This makes it harder for thieves or others who pose a threat to target you.
- **Secure room keys, IDs, and personal items**. Keep track of these items to protect your security.
- **Lock windows and doors in your room**. Secure all means of entering your space.
- **Bring a door wedge or portable door jammer for added security at night**. This provides additional security or backup if the locks on your door are insufficient.

BE AWARE OF RISKS

- **Avoid carrying or wearing expensive items**. This can reduce the risk of theft.
- **Plan for safety**. Consider potential risks and have a plan in place. Bring personal safety devices, such as whistles or alarms, and consider self-defense courses.

- **Know where emergency services are.** Locate nearby police stations and hospitals.
- **Limit social media activity.** Avoid sharing detailed travel plans until you return.
- **Use GPS tracking.** Ensure your phone and devices have tracking enabled. Share your location with a trusted contact.
- **Download offline maps.** This ensures access to navigation without data.
- **Inform someone of your travel plans.** Include your itinerary and emergency contacts.

WATCH YOUR DRINK

U.S. citizens can be targeted by criminals who add drugs to drinks to facilitate theft or assault. Drugs such as Rohypnol, ketamine, and scopolamine can cause unconsciousness. Always watch your drink and cover it if possible.

- **Meet strangers in public places.** Avoid isolated locations, such as residences or hotel rooms.
- **Do not accept drinks from strangers.** This reduces the risk of being drugged.
- **Monitor your alcohol consumption.** Be aware of any unusual symptoms.
- **If you feel unwell, seek help immediately.** Contact a trusted friend, local authorities, or the nearest U.S. Embassy or Consulate. If you are assaulted, seek medical attention and support.

Traveling abroad requires thorough preparation and awareness of potential safety and legal issues. Understanding local customs, laws, and transport options can help ensure a safe and enjoyable trip. Always stay informed and take precautions to protect yourself and your belongings.[3]

---

[3] Bureau of Consular Affairs, "Best Practices for Traveler Safety," U.S. Department of State (DOS), February 29, 2024. Available online. URL: https://travel.state.gov/content/travel/en/international-travel/before-you-go/about-our-new-products/Best-Practices-for-Traveler-Safety.html. Accessed July 30, 2024.

Section 25.2 | **Cruise Safety**

BEFORE YOUR CRUISE

- **Review the latest guidance from the Centers for Disease Control and Prevention (CDC) on cruise ship travel.**
- **Read the traveler's checklist (https://travel.state.gov/ content/travel/en/international-travel/before-you-go/ travelers-checklist.html).**
- **Check the country information pages for the countries you will visit to learn about important health and safety precautions.** Write down the contact information for the nearest U.S. Embassy or Consulate in case of an emergency.
- **Always carry your passport book with you.** You may need it for an unexpected medical evacuation or if the ship docks at an alternate port. Bring your passport even if your cruise states it is unnecessary.
- **Apply early for your passport, ensuring it will be valid for at least six months beyond your travel dates and has two or more blank pages.** Your cruise company may require you to have a passport even if U.S. Customs and Border Protection (CBP) or the foreign port of entry does not.
- **Obtain the necessary foreign visas for all stops on your cruise, even if you do not plan to disembark.**
- **Enroll in the Smart Traveler Enrollment Program (STEP) to receive important safety and security information.** For travel updates, follow @TravelGov on Twitter, Facebook, and Instagram.
- **Ensure you have medical and emergency evacuation insurance for your trip.** Consider purchasing supplemental insurance, as U.S. Medicare and Medicaid do not cover medical costs overseas.
- **Plan for unexpected travel expenses by checking with your cruise line or travel agency regarding coverage.** Verify with your health or homeowner's insurance providers and credit card companies if they offer coverage overseas. If not, consider purchasing supplemental insurance.

- **Have a contingency plan for returning home if you must remain in a foreign country longer than expected.** Make color copies of your passport photo page, foreign visas, and itinerary. Leave one copy with a trusted family member or friend and carry another separately from your actual documents. Take a photo of your travel documents with your phone for electronic copies.

MEDICATION AND VACCINATION REQUIREMENTS

- **Consult your doctor to ensure traveling abroad to your destinations is medically safe and determine if you need vaccinations or assistive devices.**
- **Check with the foreign country's embassy in the United States to confirm whether your medications are legal in each country you visit.** Learn if there are any limits or special instructions for bringing them in. For some medications, you may need a letter from your doctor, as carrying them in a prescription bottle might not suffice.
- **Ensure you have enough prescription medications to last beyond your trip dates in case of delays.** Some countries may not have equivalents of your prescription and over-the-counter (OTC) medications.
- **Carry a written copy of all your prescriptions if a country requires it, or you need to replace your medications.**

ASK YOUR CRUISE LINE

- What procedures are in place in case of an emergency.
- How family members can contact you in an emergency, including information on cell or satellite phone coverage and/or an email address for emergencies.
- What types of medical services your ship can provide, such as basic or urgent care, hospitalization, or dialysis.
- Review the cruise line's prohibited items list when packing.

DURING YOUR CRUISE

- Remember to exercise normal precautions aboard the cruise ship and onshore, as you would when traveling abroad.
- Limit your alcohol intake.
- Ensure cabin safety by keeping the door and balcony locked.
- Store travel documents and valuables securely, such as in a room safe or the ship's safe.
- If you are a crime victim, report it to the security personnel onboard. The cruise ship should have procedures for handling onboard crimes.
- Follow local laws and customs. Breaking the law may result in arrest and prosecution.
- If you are a crime victim onshore, report it to local authorities, the nearest U.S. Embassy or Consulate, and the cruise ship security personnel.
- Report a lost passport immediately to the nearest U.S. Embassy or Consulate and make plans to obtain a new passport as soon as possible.
- Follow the CDC guidance after disembarking.

OTHER THINGS TO KEEP IN MIND

- Check the travelers' page for specific issues you might face abroad, including special considerations for older travelers, those with disabilities, women, and LGBTQI+ travelers.

SPECIAL NOTES FOR TRAVEL TO CUBA

Ensure that shore excursions and purchases comply with U.S. regulations (www.state.gov/u-s-relations-with-cuba). U.S. credit and debit cards do not work in Cuba, so bring enough cash to cover your stay. This includes payments for hotels, restaurants, taxis, and souvenir shops.

Overall, ensure compliance with regulations, carry sufficient cash, and stay informed about safety, health, and legal requirements.

Taking these precautions can help ensure safe and enjoyable cruise ship travel.[1]

Section 25.3 | Charter Flights and Travel Considerations

When passengers travel by airplane, they typically take scheduled flights that operate according to prepublished schedules. However, another option is a charter flight, which differs from a scheduled flight in several key ways.

CHARTER FLIGHTS

A charter flight is not part of an airline's published schedule. For instance, an airline will not advertise a flight from Point A to Point B at 3 p.m. every Wednesday. Instead, charter flights are typically operated for specific, unscheduled itineraries. There are various types of charter flights, including:

- **Public charters**. Flights offered to the public, often as part of vacation packages.
- **Special event tours**. Charters organized for specific events like sports games or concerts.
- **Affinity (pro rata) charters**. Flights arranged by organizations for their members.
- **Single-entity charters**. Entire aircraft chartered by one entity, such as a sports team.

TRAVELING WITH A DISABILITY ON A CHARTER FLIGHT

Airlines operating charter flights must comply with the Air Carrier Access Act (ACAA) and the U.S. Department of Transportation's (DOT) disability regulations, prohibiting discrimination against air travelers with disabilities. Public charter operators (companies

---

[1] Bureau of Consular Affairs, "Cruise Ship Passengers," U.S. Department of State (DOS), March 5, 2024. Available online. URL: https://travel.state.gov/content/travel/en/international-travel/before-you-go/travelers-with-special-considerations/cruise-ship-passengers.html. Accessed July 30, 2024.

selling tickets for charter flights) must accommodate passengers with disabilities if they provide services typically offered by direct air carriers, such as check-in, gate agents, and wheelchair service.

BAGGAGE LIABILITY ON A CHARTER FLIGHT

The DOT's domestic baggage liability rules apply to all domestic charter flights operated on aircraft with more than 60 seats. These requirements are the same as those for scheduled flights. For international charter flights, the Montreal Convention applies, governing international baggage liability.

PUBLIC CHARTERS

A public charter exists when a person or company contracts for the operation of an aircraft and sells seats to the public, either directly or through travel agents. These charters often operate seasonally and as part of vacation packages, providing excellent value and frequently offering nonstop service.

Finding the Operator of Your Public Charter Flight

All sales materials must include the name of the airline operating the flight and providing the crew.

Approval of Public Charters

Ensure the public charter you book is approved by the DOT. Check the Public Charter web page (www.transportation.gov/policy/aviation-policy/licensing/public-charters) for an approved prospectus.

Signing a Contract for Public Charters

When purchasing a ticket, you must enter into an operator-participant agreement, outlining your rights. Most contracts are electronic and must be signed before travel. You are entitled to a full refund if you cancel before signing the agreement.

TARMAC DELAYS DURING PUBLIC CHARTER FLIGHTS

Tarmac delay rules apply to public charter flights at U.S. airports. The responsible party is the airline operating the aircraft and providing the crew. These rules apply only to carriers with at least one aircraft with a seating capacity of 30 or more seats.

Passenger Rights during Tarmac Delays
Rights for public charter flights are the same as for scheduled flights, including the right to disembark after a certain period.

REFUNDS DUE TO CANCELLATION OR MAJOR CHANGES
Public charter companies must notify passengers of cancellations or major changes in writing. If a charter is canceled or undergoes a major change, you are entitled to a refund. Major changes include changes in departure or return cities, dates, significant delays, hotel substitutions, or price increases exceeding 10 percent.

Right to Refund
You may cancel your trip within seven days of a major change for a full refund. If you cancel for reasons other than a major change, your right to a refund may be limited.

SPECIAL EVENT TOURS
Special event tours are public charters organized for specific events, such as sports, concerts, or cultural events. The operator must clearly state if event tickets are included.

Advertising and Pricing
Special event tour operators must have tickets in hand or a written contract for tickets at the time of sale. They can increase the tour price, but if the increase exceeds 10 percent or occurs less than 10 days before departure, participants may cancel and receive a full refund.

AFFINITY CHARTERS
Affinity charters are arranged by organizations for their members, who must pay for their airfare individually. These charters often do not carry the same consumer protection provisions as public

charters. Membership in the organization must predate the flight by six months, with certain exceptions.

Pricing and Membership Requirements

The ticket price must be uniform for all adult members, with possible discounts for children under 12.

SINGLE-ENTITY CHARTERS

Single-entity charters occur when an individual or company pays for the entire aircraft. Passengers do not pay for individual seats. For example, a sports team may charter a plane, and the team members do not pay for their seats.

Always verify the details and terms of your charter flight, including cancellation policies, refund rights, and accessibility accommodations.[1]

---

[1] "Charter Flights," U.S. Department of Transportation (DOT), March 4, 2020. Available online. URL: www.transportation.gov/individuals/aviation-consumer-protection/charter-flights. Accessed April 18, 2024.

Chapter 26 | **Hosting an International Exchange Student**

WHAT IS HOSTING?

Hosting involves bringing the world into your home, family, and community by welcoming an international high school exchange student. By hosting a student for a few weeks or an academic year, you will share cultures and form bonds that last a lifetime. These extraordinary young people, selected through highly competitive, merit-based scholarships from the U.S. Department of State, participate in programs like the Congress-Bundestag Youth Exchange (CBYX), Future Leaders Exchange (FLEX), and Youth Exchange and Study (YES) Programs. Students must maintain high academic performance, learn about American history and society, and engage in community service. Volunteer host families provide a comfortable, nurturing home, nutritious meals, and transportation to and from school activities.

HOW DO I START THE PROCESS?

To begin hosting, complete the interest form on this web page (https://eca.state.gov/programs-initiatives/host-high-school-student). A local coordinator will contact you with more information.[1]

ARE WE GOOD CANDIDATES FOR HOSTING?

Host families come in all shapes and sizes, including families with teens, no children, young children, grown children, single

---

[1] "Host a Student: Bureau of Educational and Cultural Affairs," U.S. Department of State (DOS), November 15, 2012. Available online. URL: https://eca.state.gov/programs-initiatives/host-high-school-student. Accessed July 30, 2024.

parents, and grandparents. They may live in large cities, suburban areas, farms, or small communities. A placement organization representative will help match an exchange student to your family situation.

HOW WILL OUR FAMILY BENEFIT BY HOSTING AN INTERNATIONAL EXCHANGE STUDENT?

Hosting an exchange student is a rewarding experience. You will learn about another culture and language, form a lifelong relationship with your new "son" or "daughter," and gain a friend in another country. Your family members will bond by sharing daily life with the student. Children can gain a broader perspective on the world, and young children may enjoy having an older sibling from another country. As a host family, you act as citizen diplomats, creating positive impressions about America and fostering mutual understanding and respect.

HOW LONG DO WE HAVE TO HOST OUR EXCHANGE STUDENT?

Hosting can range from serving a meal or providing an overnight stay to welcoming a student for a full academic year. You can choose to host for one semester or the entire school year.

DO I HAVE TO SEND MY SON OR DAUGHTER OVERSEAS TO HOST AN EXCHANGE STUDENT?

No. The term "exchange" refers to an exchange of cultures and ideas rather than a literal exchange of family members. However, American host siblings are welcome to apply for overseas travel.

MY FAMILY IS NOT A "TRADITIONAL" FAMILY. CAN WE STILL HOST?

Absolutely! Host families can be single parents, same-sex couples, couples without children, adoptive parents, empty nesters, military families, and more. The diversity of host families reflects the diversity of exchange students.

WHAT IS REQUIRED OF A HOST FAMILY?

Host families should provide:
- a separate bed, a suitable study area, and three meals per day
- a supportive environment as the student adjusts to a new culture
- an interest in teenagers and international students, with realistic expectations of life with a teenager
- familiarity with the local area and promotion of participation in school and community events
- a safe and secure living and learning environment

WILL MY EXCHANGE STUDENT SPEAK ENGLISH?

Yes, all students must be able to function in their classrooms in English. Proficiency levels may vary, but all students are required to speak English.

WILL I RECEIVE FINANCIAL COMPENSATION FOR HOSTING AN EXCHANGE STUDENT?

No, hosting is a volunteer opportunity. However, American host families can claim a flat $50 monthly tax deduction for the upcoming tax year.

AM I THE EXCHANGE STUDENT'S LEGAL GUARDIAN?

No, the student's natural parents remain legal guardians. The exchange program takes legal responsibility, and the student's Certificate of Health includes a medical release form for emergencies.

HOW WILL OUR EXCHANGE STUDENT GET AROUND?

Exchange students are not allowed to drive. Host families must provide transportation, whether through the school bus, family vehicle, public transportation, or biking. Host families are also responsible for transportation to school activities and events.

WHAT IF THE STUDENT NEEDS MEDICAL ATTENTION?

Exchange students are provided with health insurance that covers medical expenses. Before acceptance into the program, students undergo a physical exam and must submit a certified health report.[2]

[2] "Commonly Asked Questions," U.S. Department of State (DOS), January 8, 2013. Available online. URL: https://exchanges.state.gov/us/commonly-asked-questions-0. Accessed July 30, 2024.

Chapter 27 | **Choosing Safe Accommodations**

Choosing secure lodging in a safe area is crucial, especially when traveling alone. It is important to remember that accessibility and safety features can vary significantly worldwide and are not universal. Consider the following tips when selecting lodging for your next trip:

BEFORE YOU TRAVEL

- Research accommodations carefully. Read reviews for safety concerns. Additionally, have backup accommodations in mind.
- Arrange your first night of accommodation before you travel. If possible, arrange all accommodations in advance. You are more vulnerable when you first arrive in an unfamiliar country.
- Do not tell strangers where you are staying.
- Secure room keys, IDs (documents containing information regarding your identity), and other personal items.
- Lock windows and doors when inside your room.
- Bring a door wedge or portable door jammer to use at night.

LOCATION

- Choose a location close to transportation and public services.
- Be aware of the crime rates in the area where your lodging is located.

- Check for special accommodations if needed, such as a working elevator and ramps.

24-HOUR RECEPTION
- Contact the front desk if you notice suspicious behavior.
- Consider hotels with gate access, guards, and other security measures if appropriate.
- Meet visitors in the lobby.
- Carry your room key separately from the key packet with your room number.

YOUR ROOM
- Upon arrival, scan your room. Check behind curtains, under the bed, and other places to ensure it is safe.
- Check that phones work.
- Look for carbon monoxide detectors, fire alarms, and fire extinguishers.
- Confirm that all external doors, windows, and bathrooms have functioning locks.
- Ensure curtains provide adequate privacy.
- Check for odd-looking electronics that might indicate hidden cameras. Do not tamper with these.
- Report any issues to the front desk immediately.

THE SAFEST FLOOR
Travel industry experts recommend choosing a room located above the first floor, ideally between the third and sixth floors. These floors are high enough to avoid easy break-ins but low enough for safe evacuation in case of a fire.

CLOSE TO AN EMERGENCY EXIT
- Review the emergency plan posted in your room.
- Locate the closest emergency exit and familiarize yourself with the route upon arrival.

- Be aware that exiting through a window may not be an option.[1]

BE AWARE OF RISKS

- To prevent theft, avoid carrying or wearing anything expensive.
- Use your best judgment to avoid unsafe situations. Think ahead and devise a safety plan. Consider bringing personal safety whistles/alarms and taking self-defense courses before you travel.
- Find out where emergency services, like police stations and hospitals, are located nearby in case of an emergency.
- Do not share detailed travel information on social media until you return.
- Ensure your phone and other personal devices have a "find my phone" or similar Global Positioning System (GPS) tracker for emergencies. Consider sharing your location with a trusted contact back home.
- Download map applications that work with GPS instead of data to ensure access to local maps and routes. Keep your mobile device charged.
- Tell someone you trust back home about your travel plans. Include where you will stay, any distant destinations, and an emergency contact.[2]

---

[1] Bureau of Consular Affairs, "Lodging Safety," U.S. Department of State (DOS), February 14, 2024. Available online. URL: https://travel.state.gov/content/travel/en/international-travel/before-you-go/lodging-safety.html. Accessed July 30, 2024.
[2] Bureau of Consular Affairs, "Best Practices for Traveler Safety," U.S. Department of State (DOS), February 14, 2024. Available online. URL: https://travel.state.gov/content/travel/en/international-travel/before-you-go/about-our-new-products/Best-Practices-for-Traveler-Safety.html. Accessed July 30, 2024.

Chapter 28 | **Hotel Safety and Security Concerns**

BOOKING A HOTEL: BEWARE OF SCAMS

When planning a hotel stay for a summer vacation, it is essential to be aware of potential scams that could target travelers. Scammers often try to take advantage of people in unfamiliar surroundings. Here are some common scams to watch out for:

The Late-Night Call from the Front Desk

You may receive a late-night call from someone claiming to be from the front desk, stating there is a problem with your credit card and requesting you to verify the number over the phone. This is likely a scam. If a hotel genuinely has an issue with your card, they will ask you to visit the front desk in person.

The Pizza Delivery Deal

Another scam involves finding a pizza delivery flyer slipped under your hotel door. When you call to order, they ask for your credit card number over the phone. However, the flyer could be fake, and a scammer could now have your information. Before ordering, verify the business or get recommendations from the front desk.

The Fake Wi-Fi Network

Scammers may set up fake Wi-Fi networks with names similar to the hotel's. Using these networks can give scammers access to your personal information. Always check with the hotel to confirm the authorized network before connecting.[1]

---

[1] "The Hazards of Hoteling," Federal Trade Commission (FTC), July 1, 2014. Available online. URL: www.military-consumer.gov/scam-alerts/hazards-hoteling. Accessed July 30, 2024.

RENTAL LISTING SCAMS

Scammers also target travelers looking for apartments or vacation rentals. They create fake rental listings designed to grab your attention and money before you realize the property does not exist or is not available.

How Rental Scam Ads Work

Scammers often take over legitimate rental listings, copy the pictures and descriptions, and replace the contact information with their own. They post these fake ads on various websites. When you reach out, the scammer may ask for an application fee, deposit, first month's rent, or vacation rental charge. Once they have your money, they disappear, leaving you without a place to stay.

WHAT TO DO

- **Search online for the rental location's address and the property owner or rental company's name**. If other ads list the same address but different owners, it could be a scam.
- **Verify the rental listing on the official website of the rental company**. If the property is not listed there, it might be a scam.

Scammers Create Listings for Nonexistent Properties

Scammers may create listings for properties that are not for rent or do not exist, often offering surprisingly low rent or amazing amenities. They may claim to be out of the country and push for a quick decision. They might ask for payment via wire transfer, gift card, or cryptocurrency, promising to send keys immediately. After payment, the scammer disappears.

WHAT TO DO

- **Do not send a payment for a property you have never seen or to someone you have never met**. Payment via wire transfer, gift card, or cryptocurrency is often irretrievable. If you cannot see the property or sign a lease in person, continue looking for other options.

Evaluating Rental Listings

- **Search online for the property owner or rental company's name with keywords such as "complaint," "review," or "scam" to learn about others' experiences.**
- **Consider the price of the rental**. If the rent is much lower than others in the area, it might be a scam. Beware of pressure to quickly decide on a "great deal."
- **Inspect the property in person or request a virtual tour**. Verify the rental agent's credentials and confirm the property owner through official records.

PROTECT YOUR PERSONAL INFORMATION AND MONEY

- **Never share personal or financial information with anyone who contacts you claiming to be associated with the owner or rental company**. Always use verified contact details.
- **Avoid paying with cash, wire transfers, gift cards, or cryptocurrency**. Once sent, these payment methods are often irretrievable. If anyone insists on these payment methods, it is likely a scam.

REPORTING PROBLEMS

If you encounter a rental listing scam, report it to:
- local law enforcement and the website where the ad was posted
- the FTC at https://reportfraud.ftc.gov
- your state attorney general via www.consumerresources.org/file-a-complaint[2]

---

[2] "Rental Listing Scams," Federal Trade Commission (FTC), August 2022. Available online. URL: https://consumer.ftc.gov/articles/rental-listing-scams. Accessed July 30, 2024.

Part 5 | **Pretravel Preparations**

Chapter 29 | U.S. Passport Essentials

Chapter Contents

Section 29.1 | How to Apply for a U.S. Passport

ELIGIBILITY TO GET A PASSPORT
If you are unable to renew your U.S. passport or if this is your first passport, you must apply for a new one. To be eligible, you must be either a U.S. citizen by birth or naturalization or a qualifying U.S. noncitizen national.

You must apply in person at a passport acceptance facility, as the process cannot be completed online or by mail.

ITEMS YOU NEED TO APPLY FOR A PASSPORT
Application Form (DS-11)
- You can complete Form DS-11 online and print it, download it, and complete it by hand, or pick it up at your local passport acceptance facility or regional agency.
- Do not sign Form DS-11 until instructed to do so by the passport acceptance official at your appointment.

Personal Documents
- original proof of citizenship
- an acceptable photo ID
- a photocopy of both your citizenship document and photo ID

Passport Photo
- a recent passport-style photo that meets the required specifications

Passport Fee
- Pay the required fee, which may vary depending on the type of passport and processing speed.

Application Submission
- You must apply in person at a passport acceptance facility, such as a library or post office. Some facilities require

appointments or have limited hours. You can find your nearest facility (https://iafdb.travel.state.gov).

IF YOU NEED YOUR PASSPORT QUICKLY

For emergency or urgent travel, or if you require expedited processing, you can learn how and where to get your passport quickly (https://travel.state.gov/content/travel/en/passports/get-fast.html). The processing time may vary throughout the year, and additional fees may apply. Use the fee calculator or chart (https://travel.state.gov/content/travel/en/passports/how-apply/fees.html) to determine the cost.

IF YOU ARE OUTSIDE THE UNITED STATES

Contact the U.S. Embassy or Consulate near you to request a passport while you are outside the United States.

IF YOU NEED TO CHANGE YOUR NAME OR CORRECT YOUR NEW PASSPORT

If you change your name or find an error in your passport, you will need an updated passport. The process, cost, and required forms depend on how long you have had your passport. Follow the steps provided by the U.S. Department of State (https://travel.state.gov/content/travel/en/passports/have-passport/change-correct.html) to change your name or correct your passport.

CHECK THE STATUS OF YOUR PASSPORT APPLICATION

To check the status of your passport application, follow the steps outlined by the U.S. Department of State (https://travel.state.gov/content/travel/en/passports/need-passport/status.html).[1]

---

[1] "Apply for a New Adult Passport," USA.gov, December 6, 2023. Available online. URL: www.usa.gov/apply-adult-passport. Accessed July 30, 2024.

Section 29.2 | **Renewing Your U.S. Passport**

DETERMINE IF YOU CAN RENEW YOUR PASSPORT

If any of the following conditions apply, you cannot renew your U.S. passport and must instead apply for a new passport in person using Form DS-11:

- The passport was issued before your 16th birthday.
- The passport was issued more than 15 years ago.
- The passport is damaged, lost, or stolen. Learn how to report it.
- The passport was issued in your previous name, and you do not have a legal document, such as a marriage license, to prove your legal name change.

If none of the above situations apply, you can renew your U.S. passport.

HOW TO RENEW YOUR PASSPORT AND THE DOCUMENTS YOU WILL NEED

Passports can only be renewed by mail, as online renewals are currently paused. Since it can take up to three months to process your application, it is crucial to renew your passport before it expires.

To renew your passport, you will typically need the following items:

- **Application form (DS-82)**. You can fill out Form DS-82 online, download and fill it out by hand, or pick up a copy from your local passport acceptance facility or regional agency.
- **Passport photo**. A recent passport-style photo that meets the required specifications.
- **Passport fee**. The required fee for passport renewal.
- **Most recent passport**. Submit your current passport with your renewal application.
- **Name change documentation (if applicable)**. If your name has changed, provide legal documentation, such as a marriage certificate.

Learn how to submit all your documentation and passport fees by mail (https://travel.state.gov/content/travel/en/passports/have-passport/renew.html).

BE AWARE OF PASSPORT EXPIRATION RULES FOR YOUR DESTINATION

Some countries and airlines will not allow a U.S. passport holder to enter if their passport expires in less than six months.

To check your destination country's U.S. passport expiration rules, visit the U.S. Department of State's (DOS) country information page (https://travel.state.gov/content/travel/en/international-travel/International-Travel-Country-Information-Pages.html). On the left side, search for the country name in the "learn about your destination" box. On that country's page, look for the "passport validity" section.[1]

Section 29.3 | Getting a Passport for a Minor

Most children must appear in person at a passport acceptance facility to apply for a passport. The cost will vary depending on the child's age.

CHILDREN UNDER 16

All children under 16 must appear in person to apply. A parent (preferably both) must be present and sign the passport application. Follow the step-by-step process for children under 16 from the State Department (https://travel.state.gov/content/travel/en/passports/need-passport/under-16.html) to ensure you have the proper forms and documents. One step will help you determine the passport fee.

---

[1] "Renew an Adult Passport," USA.gov, December 6, 2023. Available online. URL: www.usa.gov/renew-adult-passport. Accessed July 30, 2024.

You cannot renew your child's passport. If your child is under 16 and their passport has expired or will expire soon, you must submit a new application in person.

CHILDREN AGED 16–17

Children aged 16–17 can apply for passports alone if they have their identification documents. A parent must either provide a signed statement acknowledging they are aware the child is seeking a passport or attend the passport appointment with them.

Follow the step-by-step process from the State Department (https://travel.state.gov/content/travel/en/passports/need-pass-port/16-17.html) to ensure you have the proper forms. One step will help you determine the passport fee.

Children aged 16–17 cannot renew their passport if it was issued before they turned 16. Instead, they must submit an application in person for a new passport.

CHILDREN IN CUSTODY DISPUTES

If you are concerned that your child may be taken abroad by the other parent without your knowledge, you can enroll them in the Children's Passport Issuance Alert Program (CPIAP; https://travel.state.gov/content/travel/en/International-Parental-Child-Abduction/prevention/passport-issuance-alert-program.html).

IF YOU NEED YOUR CHILD'S PASSPORT QUICKLY

Depending on when and why your child is traveling, you may need to use the expedited process (https://travel.state.gov/content/travel/en/passports/get-fast.html). The processing time varies throughout the year, and there may be additional fees. Use the fee calculator or chart for more information.

IF YOU AND YOUR CHILD ARE OUTSIDE THE UNITED STATES

If you are outside the United States, contact the U.S. Embassy or Consulate near you to request a passport (https://travel.state.gov/content/travel/en/passports/need-passport/outside-us.html).

CHECK THE STATUS OF YOUR CHILD'S PASSPORT APPLICATION

Follow the steps from the Department of State (DOS; https://travel.state.gov/content/travel/en/passports/need-passport/status.html) to check the status of your child's passport application or renewal online.

BE AWARE OF PASSPORT EXPIRATION RULES FOR YOUR DESTINATION

Some countries and airlines will not allow a U.S. passport holder to enter if their passport expires in less than six months.

Check your destination country's U.S. passport expiration rules on the DOS's country information page (https://travel.state.gov/content/travel/en/international-travel/International-Travel-Country-Information-Pages.html). On the left, search for the country name in the "Learn About Your Destination" box. On that country's page, look for the "Passport Validity" section.[1]

---

[1] "Get a Passport for a Minor under 18," USA.gov, December 18, 2023. Available online. URL: www.usa.gov/child-passport. Accessed July 30, 2024.

Chapter 30 | Insurance and Financial Protection for Travelers

IMPORTANCE OF INSURANCE FOR TRAVELERS
Severe illness or injury abroad can impose a significant financial burden on travelers. Regardless of whether they have a domestic health insurance plan, travelers can substantially reduce their out-of-pocket costs for medical care received abroad by purchasing specialized insurance policies before their trip. Three types of policies—travel insurance, travel health insurance, and medical evacuation insurance—each provide different types of coverage for illness or injury. Such policies are particularly beneficial for travelers with preexisting medical conditions. In addition to cost protection, these insurance options can help travelers obtain medical care abroad.

Basic accident or travel health insurance might be necessary for travelers with certain itineraries. For example, although cruise lines employ health-care staff, the cost of medical treatment delivered onboard a ship may not be included in the price of a passenger's ticket. Therefore, travelers on cruise ships should consider investing in specialized insurance policies.

DOMESTIC HEALTH INSURANCE AND OVERSEAS TRAVEL
Some U.S. health insurance carriers cover medical emergencies that occur when policyholders travel internationally. Travelers should contact their insurer before traveling to learn what medical services, if any, their policies cover.

269

Suggested questions to ask before purchasing a supplemental travel health insurance policy:

- Coverage requirements:
  - Do you need preauthorization before receiving treatment, hospital admission, or other medical services?
  - Is a second opinion required before receiving emergency treatment?
  - What are the policies regarding care received "out of network"?
  - Does the company provide access to a 24/7/365 physician-backed support center?
- Potential exclusions:
  - Does the policy cover injuries from high-risk activities (e.g., skydiving, scuba diving, mountain climbing)?
  - Does the policy cover mental health (psychiatric) emergencies?
- Preexisting medical conditions:
  - Does the policy cover exacerbations of preexisting medical conditions?
  - Does the policy cover pregnancy complications or neonatal intensive care (NICU)?

TRAVEL INSURANCE

Travel insurance protects the traveler's financial investment in a trip, covering aspects such as lost baggage and trip cancellation. Travelers who become ill before departure may avoid or postpone travel if their financial investment is protected. However, travel insurance may not cover medical expenses abroad, so travelers should carefully research coverage and consider additional travel health and medical evacuation insurance.

SUPPLEMENTAL TRAVEL HEALTH AND MEDICAL EVACUATION INSURANCE

Travel health insurance and medical evacuation insurance are short-term supplemental policies covering health-care costs abroad.

Travelers can purchase these policies separately or together. Key features to consider include whether the insurer guarantees direct hospital payment, offers 24-hour physician-backed support, provides emergency medical transport, and covers high-risk activities.

In some cases, medical evacuation (medevac) from a resource-poor area to a hospital delivering definitive care may be necessary. The cost of medevac varies by location, ranging from $25,000 within North America to $250,000 for remote locations. Costs increase with the severity of the patient's condition. Medevac insurance covers transportation costs, including to another country if needed.

FINDING AN INSURANCE PROVIDER

Several organizations provide information about purchasing travel health and medical evacuation insurance, including the U.S. Department of State (DOS), International Association for Medical Assistance to Travelers (IAMAT), U.S. Travel Insurance Association (UStiA), and the American Association of Retired Persons (AARP). The Centers for Disease Control and Prevention (CDC) does not endorse any provider or medical insurance company.

TRAVELERS WITH UNDERLYING MEDICAL CONDITIONS

Travelers with underlying medical conditions should discuss their concerns with the insurer before departure. In some cases, insurance companies may not cover claims due to preexisting conditions or poor documentation of expenses. Travelers should store copies of their health records with a medical assistance company, obtain letters from health-care providers detailing medical conditions and medications (including generic names), and pack medications in their original packaging in carry-on luggage. Travelers with known heart conditions should carry a recent electrocardiogram (ECG or EKG) copy.

MEDICARE BENEFICIARIES

Medicare beneficiaries should carefully examine their coverage and supplement it with additional travel health insurance. Except in limited circumstances, Medicare does not cover medical costs outside the United States or medical evacuation. Medigap plans C,

D, F, G, M, and N cover some emergency care outside the United States. After meeting the $250 yearly deductible, these plans pay 80 percent of emergency care costs during the first 60 days of international travel, with a lifetime maximum of $50,000. More information on Medicare and Medigap options is available at Medicare.gov (www.medicare.gov/supplements-other-insurance/medigap-travel).

PAYING FOR HEALTH SERVICES RECEIVED ABROAD

During the pretravel consultation, discuss insurance options and suggest that all travelers consider purchasing supplemental medical insurance coverage, particularly if traveling to remote destinations or places lacking high-quality medical facilities. Strongly encourage supplemental medical insurance coverage for travelers planning extended international travel, those with underlying health conditions, and those participating in high-risk activities (e.g., scuba diving, mountain climbing) abroad. Travel health insurers can assist in organizing and coordinating care and keeping relatives informed in case of a medical emergency.

Nationalized health-care services at a destination may not cover the costs for nonresidents. Even with a supplemental travel health insurance policy, receiving medical care abroad usually requires cash or credit card payment at the point of service, potentially leading to significant expenses. U.S. citizens paying for health-care abroad should obtain copies of all charges and receipts and, if necessary, contact a U.S. consular officer for assistance with transferring funds from the United States.

The U.S. Department of State (DOS) may offer limited emergency medical assistance loans to U.S. citizens who experience a medical emergency abroad but cannot pay at the point of service or arrange for funds transfer. Travelers must repay these loans. Once issued, the DOS will limit the traveler's U.S. passport and, in most cases, will not issue a new passport until the loan is paid in full. U.S. citizens should contact the nearest U.S. Embassy or Consulate, or the DOS Office of Overseas Citizens Services (OCS), at 888-407-4747 (or from abroad, 202-501-4444) for information about assistance options and eligibility requirements.

TRAVEL MEDICINE PROFESSIONAL RESPONSIBILITIES

- Assess travelers' health profiles, including underlying medical conditions.
- Identify potential medical needs abroad, including health risks based on itinerary, destination, travel duration, transportation method, accommodations, and planned activities.
- Review domestic health policies to identify gaps in coverage for potential medical needs.
- Discuss supplemental insurance types (travel, travel health, and medical evacuation) and help choose policies that cover potential medical needs abroad.
- Advise travelers on steps to take if they require medical care abroad, including paying out-of-pocket and submitting bills for reimbursement.

TRAVELER RESPONSIBILITIES

Before Travel

- Review domestic health insurance policies to understand overseas coverage.
- Purchase supplemental travel health insurance based on potential medical needs and risks.
- Identify medical service providers at the destination, including directories of English-speaking health-care providers (see International Association for Medical Assistance to Travelers (IAMAT; www.iamat.org)).
- Confirm with the insurance company that they reimburse out-of-pocket payments made to health-care providers abroad. Travelers should plan to pay for services upfront with cash or credit card.

During Travel

- Carry insurance policy identity cards and insurance claim forms.
- Have contact information for medical providers at the destination.

273

- Keep copies of all charges and receipts for medical care received.

After Travel
- Seek medical attention promptly upon returning to the United States at the first sign of any unexpected complications.
- Bring copies of all summary records, charges, and receipts for medical care received abroad.
- Provide U.S. health-care providers with travel details, including dates, medical care received, and contact information for international health-care providers.[1]

---

[1] "Travel Insurance, Travel Health Insurance, and Medical Evacuation Insurance," Centers for Disease Control and Prevention (CDC), May 1, 2023. Available online. URL: wwwnc.cdc.gov/travel/yellowbook/2024/health-care-abroad/insurance. Accessed July 30, 2024.

Chapter 31 | Vaccination Recommendations

Chapter Contents

Section 31.1 | Vaccines for Travelers

Vaccines protect travelers from serious diseases. Depending on where you travel, you may come into contact with rare diseases in the United States, such as yellow fever. Some vaccines may also be required for travel to certain destinations.

Getting vaccinated will help keep you safe and healthy during your travels. It will also help ensure that you do not bring any serious diseases home to your family, friends, and community.

WHICH VACCINES DO I NEED BEFORE TRAVELING?

The vaccines you need before traveling depend on several factors, including:

- **Destination**. Some countries require proof of vaccination for certain diseases, such as yellow fever or polio. Traveling to developing countries and rural areas may expose you to more diseases, necessitating additional vaccines before your visit.
- **Health status**. If you are pregnant, have an ongoing illness, or have a weakened immune system, you may need additional vaccines.
- **Previous vaccinations**. It is important to be up-to-date on your routine vaccinations. While diseases such as measles are rare in the United States, they are more common in other countries.

HOW FAR IN ADVANCE SHOULD I GET VACCINATED BEFORE TRAVELING?

It is essential to get vaccinated at least four to six weeks before your trip. This timeframe allows the vaccines to take effect, ensuring protection during travel. It also provides sufficient time for any vaccines that require multiple doses.

TRAVELING WITH A CHILD

Make sure they get the measles vaccine. Measles remains common in some countries. Vaccinating your child will protect them from measles and prevent the disease's spread upon returning to the United States.

WHERE CAN I GET TRAVEL VACCINES?

You can obtain travel vaccines from the following:

- travel clinic (www.istm.org/AF_CstmClinicDirectory.asp)
- health department (www.naccho.org/membership/lhd-directory)
- yellow fever vaccination clinic (wwwnc.cdc.gov/travel/page/search-for-stamaril-clinics)
- other vaccines (www.vaccines.gov/search)[1]

Examples of Vaccines

Here is a list of possible vaccines that you may need for the first time or as boosters before you travel:

- chickenpox
- cholera
- coronavirus 2019 (COVID-19)
- flu (influenza)
- hepatitis A
- hepatitis B
- Japanese encephalitis
- MMR (measles, mumps, rubella)
- meningococcal
- pneumococcal
- polio
- rabies
- shingles
- Tdap (tetanus, diphtheria, pertussis)
- typhoid
- yellow fever[2]

---

[1] "Vaccines for Travelers," U.S. Department of Health and Human Services (HHS), April 29, 2021. Available online. URL: www.hhs.gov/immunization/who-and-when/travel/index.html. Accessed July 31, 2024.

[2] "Need Travel Vaccines? Plan Ahead," Centers for Disease Control and Prevention (CDC), January 13, 2023. Available online. URL: wwwnc.cdc.gov/travel/page/travel-vaccines. Accessed July 31, 2024.

WHAT RESOURCES CAN I USE TO PREPARE FOR MY TRIP?

Consider these resources while planning your trip:

- Visit the Centers for Disease Control and Prevention's (CDC) travel website (wwwnc.cdc.gov/travel) to find out which vaccines you may need based on your destination, activities, and health conditions.
- Download the CDC's Vaccine Schedules app (www.cdc.gov/vaccines/hcp/imz-schedules/app. html) to find recommended vaccines for children and adults, categorized by age group and medical conditions.
- Check the current travel notices (wwwnc.cdc.gov/travel/notices) to stay informed about any new disease outbreaks or vaccine recommendations for your destination.
- Visit the State Department's website (https://travel. state.gov/content/travel/en/international-travel/before-you-go/your-health-abroad.html) to learn about vaccinations, insurance, and medical emergencies while traveling.

Ensuring you are properly vaccinated before traveling is crucial for your health and safety. By preparing well in advance, you can protect yourself from various diseases and avoid bringing infections back to your community. Consult with your health-care provider to discuss the necessary vaccines and precautions for your trip.[3]

Section 31.2 | Routine Vaccinations for Travelers

WHAT ARE ROUTINE VACCINES?

Routine vaccines are recommended for everyone in the United States based on age and vaccine history. While most people consider

---

[3] See footnote [1].

these as childhood vaccines received before starting school, there are also routine vaccines for adolescents and adults.

WHY ARE ROUTINE VACCINES IMPORTANT FOR TRAVELERS?

Since most U.S. children receive routine vaccines, many vaccine-preventable diseases, such as measles, mumps, or chickenpox, are uncommon in the United States. However, international travel can increase the chances of contracting and spreading diseases not common domestically. Popular destinations, including Europe, continue to experience outbreaks of measles and other vaccine-preventable diseases.

Ensure you are up-to-date on all your routine vaccines (wwwnc. cdc.gov/travel/page/routine-vaccines). These vaccinations protect against infectious diseases that can spread rapidly in groups of unvaccinated people. While many of these diseases are uncommon in the United States, they are still prevalent in other countries.

Check the Centers for Disease Control and Prevention's (CDC) website (wwwnc.cdc.gov/travel/destinations/list) for your destination to determine the necessary vaccines or medicines and understand the diseases or health risks there.

Make an appointment with your health-care provider or a travel health specialist (wwwnc.cdc.gov/travel/page/find-clinic) at least one month before departure. They can help you obtain destination-specific vaccines, medicines, and information. Discussing your health concerns, itinerary, and planned activities with your provider allows for tailored advice and recommendations.

WHAT ROUTINE VACCINES DO YOU NEED?

The routine vaccines you need before travel may depend on your age, health, and vaccine history. You may require an accelerated dose or a booster dose before traveling.

Routine vaccinations related to travel may include the following:
- coronavirus (COVID-19)
- chickenpox (varicella)
- hepatitis A
- hepatitis B

- human papillomavirus (HPV)
- influenza
- measles, mumps, rubella (MMR)
- meningococcal
- pneumococcal
- polio
- rotavirus
- tetanus, diphtheria, pertussis (Tdap)
- shingles (zoster)

Staying current with routine vaccines is crucial for protecting yourself and others during travel. These vaccinations help prevent the spread of infectious diseases and safeguard public health.[1]

Section 31.3 | Yellow Fever Vaccine

A safe and effective yellow fever vaccine has been available for more than 80 years. The vaccine, a live attenuated form of the virus, is administered as a single injection and provides lifelong protection for most individuals. It is recommended for people aged nine months or older who are traveling to or living in areas at risk for yellow fever in Africa and South America. Additionally, some countries require proof of vaccination for entry.

YELLOW FEVER VACCINE RECOMMENDATIONS
For most individuals, a single dose of the yellow fever vaccine provides long-lasting protection, eliminating the need for a booster dose. However, travelers heading to regions with ongoing outbreaks may consider getting a booster dose if it has been 10 years or more since their last vaccination. Some countries may also mandate a

[1] "Routine Vaccines," Centers for Disease Control and Prevention (CDC), January 31, 2022. Available online. URL: wwwnc.cdc.gov/travel/page/routine-vaccines. Accessed July 31, 2024.

booster dose; travelers should check specific country requirements on the Centers for Disease Control and Prevention's (CDC)
Yellow Book web page (wwwnc.cdc.gov/travel/yellowbook/2024/
preparing/yellow-fever-vaccine-malaria-prevention-by-country/
brazil#seldyfm879).

Consult with your health-care provider to determine if you need
an initial or booster yellow fever vaccination before traveling to
at-risk areas.

INCREASED RISK OF VACCINE REACTIONS

Certain individuals may have an increased risk of adverse reactions
to the yellow fever vaccine but may still benefit from vaccination.
These individuals, or their guardians, should consult with a health-
care provider:

- infants aged six to eight months
- individuals over 60 years old
- pregnant women
- breastfeeding women

CONTRAINDICATIONS FOR THE YELLOW FEVER VACCINE

The yellow fever vaccine is not recommended for certain individuals, including those who:

- are allergic to any component of the vaccine (such as
  eggs)
- are under six months of age
- have received an organ transplant
- have been diagnosed with a malignant tumor
- have a thymus disorder associated with abnormal
  immune function
- have a primary immunodeficiency
- are using immunosuppressive or immunomodulatory
  therapies
- have symptoms of HIV infection or a CD4+
  T-lymphocyte count less than 200/mm^3 (or less than
  15% of total lymphocytes in children aged six years or
  younger)

It is important to distinguish between the CDC's vaccine recommendations and country entry requirements. Proof of yellow fever vaccination may be mandatory for entry into certain countries.

REACTIONS TO YELLOW FEVER VACCINE

Reactions to the yellow fever vaccine are generally mild and may include headaches, muscle aches, and low-grade fevers. Rarely, severe reactions can occur, including:

- anaphylaxis (severe allergic reaction causing difficulty breathing or swallowing)
- encephalitis or meningitis (inflammation of the brain, spinal cord, or surrounding tissues)
- Guillain-Barré syndrome (GBS; an uncommon neurological disorder causing muscle weakness and sometimes paralysis)
- internal organ dysfunction or failure

If you develop symptoms such as fever, headache, tiredness, body aches, vomiting, or diarrhea after receiving the vaccine, consult your health-care provider.

YELLOW FEVER VACCINE, PREGNANCY, AND CONCEPTION

Many pregnant women have been administered the yellow fever vaccine without apparent adverse effects on the fetus. However, as a live virus vaccine, it carries a theoretical risk. Pregnant women should avoid or postpone travel to areas where yellow fever is risky. If travel cannot be avoided, vaccination should be discussed with a health-care provider.

A two-week delay between vaccination and conception is generally considered adequate, although a one-month delay is sometimes recommended as a more conservative approach. If a woman is vaccinated during pregnancy, significant problems are unlikely, and the baby is expected to be born healthy.[1]

---

[1] "Yellow Fever Vaccine," Centers for Disease Control and Prevention (CDC), May 15, 2024. Available online. URL: www.cdc.gov/yellow-fever/vaccine. Accessed July 30, 2024.

Chapter 32 | Travel Health Kits for International Travelers

International travelers, regardless of their destination, should assemble and carry a travel health kit. The contents should be tailored to specific needs, the type and length of travel, and the destination(s). Kits can be assembled at home or purchased at a local store, pharmacy, or online. Travel health kits ensure travelers have the necessary supplies to manage preexisting medical conditions, prevent illness and injury related to traveling, and address minor health issues as they arise.

TRAVELING WITH MEDICATIONS

International travelers should carry all medications in their original containers with clear labels that identify the contents, the patient's name, and dosing information. While travelers may prefer using small bags, pillboxes, or daily-dose containers, officials at ports of entry may require medications to be in their original prescription containers.

Travelers should also carry copies of all prescriptions, including generic names, ideally translated into the local language of the destination. For controlled substances and injectable medications, a note on letterhead from the prescribing clinician or travel clinic is necessary. Translating the letter into the local language of the destination and attaching it to the original document can be helpful if needed during the trip. Some countries do not permit certain medications. Travelers should contact the U.S. Embassy or Consulate of the destination country for questions about medication restrictions, especially concerning controlled substances.

A travel health kit is only useful if it is easily accessible. Travelers should always carry the kit with them (e.g., in a carry-on bag); however, sharp objects like scissors and fine splinter tweezers must remain in checked luggage. Travelers should ensure that any liquid or gel-based items in carry-on bags do not exceed size limits, although exceptions are made for certain medical reasons. For more information, contact the Transportation Security Administration (TSA) or visit their customer service web page. The U.S. Embassy or Consulate at the destination can also provide details.

SUPPLIES FOR PREEXISTING MEDICAL CONDITIONS
Travelers with preexisting medical conditions should bring enough medication for the duration of the trip and an extra supply in case of unforeseen extensions. If additional supplies or medications are needed for managing exacerbations of existing conditions, these should also be packed. Travelers with conditions such as allergies or diabetes should consider wearing an alert bracelet. It may be challenging to purchase needles and syringes in some locations, so travelers should bring more than needed. Additionally, those needing needles and syringes must carry a letter from the prescribing clinician on letterhead.

GENERAL TRAVEL HEALTH KIT SUPPLIES
The following is a list of items travelers should consider including in a basic travel health kit. Ensure travelers have details and instructions for any prescribed medications, including antibiotics for self-treatment of diarrhea, medications for altitude illness, and malaria chemoprophylaxis.

Prescription Medications and Medical Supplies
- antibiotics for self-treatment of moderate to severe travelers' diarrhea (if prescribed)
- antihistamines, epinephrine autoinjectors (e.g., an EpiPen 2-Pak), short course of oral steroid medications (for travelers,

including children, with a history of severe allergic reactions or anaphylaxis)
- antimalarial medication (if prescribed)
- insulin and diabetes testing supplies
- medicine to prevent or treat altitude illness (if prescribed)
- needles or syringes (plus extras) for injectable medicines
- prescription glasses/contact lenses (consider packing an extra pair of each)
- prescription medicines taken regularly at home
- sleep aids (if prescribed)

Pack all prescription medicines and necessary medical supplies in a carry-on bag. Medicines should be in their original containers with labels clearly identifying the contents, patient name, and dosing information. Consider wearing a medical alert bracelet or necklace if you have chronic illnesses or underlying health conditions.

Over-the-Counter Medications
- over-the-counter (OTC) medicines taken regularly at home
- medicines for pain or fever, such as acetaminophen, aspirin, and ibuprofen
- medicines for stomach upset or diarrhea, such as antidiarrheal medication (e.g., loperamide (Imodium) or bismuth subsalicylate (Pepto-Bismol)), packets of oral rehydration salts for dehydration, mild laxatives, and antacids
- medicines for mild upper respiratory conditions, such as antihistamines, decongestants (alone or in combination with antihistamines), cough suppressants or expectorants, and cough drops
- medicines for motion sickness
- sleep aids (nonprescription)
- eye drops
- nose drops or spray

Basic First Aid Items
- adhesive bandages and tape (multiple sizes)
- antifungal and antibacterial spray or creams

- anti-itch gel or cream for insect bites and stings
- antiseptic wound cleanser
- commercial suture kit (for travel to remote areas)
- cotton swabs
- digital thermometer
- disposable latex-free gloves
- elastic/compression bandage wrap for sprains and strains
- first aid quick reference card
- gauze
- hydrocortisone cream (1%)
- moleskin or molefoam for blister prevention and treatment
- safety pins
- scissors (pack sharp metal objects in checked baggage; small, rounded-tip bandage scissors may be available for purchase in certain stores or online)
- triangular bandage to wrap injuries and to make an arm or shoulder sling
- tweezers (pack sharp metal objects in checked baggage)

Supplies to Prevent Illness and Injury

- antibacterial hand wipes or an alcohol-based hand sanitizer containing greater than or equal to 60 percent alcohol
- earplugs
- face masks
- insect repellents for skin and clothing
- latex condoms
- mosquito net (for protection against insect bites while sleeping; can be pretreated with insect repellent)
- personal safety equipment (e.g., child safety seats, bicycle or motorcycle helmets)
- sun protection (e.g., protective clothing, sunglasses, sunscreen)
- water purification method(s) if visiting remote areas, camping, or staying in areas where access to clean water is limited

Documents

- contact information card (carry at all times) that includes the street addresses, telephone numbers, and email addresses of:
  - family member or close contact remaining in the United States
  - health-care provider(s) at home
  - hospitals or clinics (including emergency services) at your destination(s)
  - insurance policy information
  - lodging at the destination(s)
  - U.S. Embassy or Consulate address and telephone number in your destination country or countries
- copies of all prescriptions for medications, eyeglasses/contacts, and other medical supplies, including generic names; preferably translated into the local language of the destination
- documentation of preexisting conditions (e.g., diabetes or allergies) in English and preferably translated into the local language of the destination
- electrocardiogram (ECG or EKG) if you have existing heart disease, including any known "abnormal heart rhythms" (arrhythmias)
- health insurance, supplemental travel health insurance, medical evacuation insurance, and travel insurance policy numbers; carrier contact information; and copies of claim forms
- International Certificate of Vaccination or Prophylaxis (ICVP) card showing proof of vaccination, or an appropriate medical waiver, for travel to destinations where vaccinations are required for entry

In addition to bringing the medical documents on this list, leave copies with a family member or close contact who will remain in the United States in case of an emergency. Consider having electronic copies of documents as well.

TRAVEL KITS WHEN TRAVELING WITH CHILDREN

The following is a checklist of items travelers might consider bringing while traveling with children.

Supplies for Children

- baby wipes
- change mat
- children's medicine for pain or fever
- diapers
- insect repellent (avoid using products containing oil of lemon eucalyptus (OLE) or para-menthane-3,8-diol (PMD) on children under 3 years old)
- medicines taken regularly at home
- motor vehicle restraints (e.g., stroller, seatbelts, or car seat)
- rash cream
- sterilizing equipment for baby bottles
- sun protection
- thermometer

COMMERCIAL MEDICAL KITS

Travelers can obtain commercial medical kits for various circumstances, from basic first aid to advanced emergency life support. Companies also manufacture advanced medical kits for adventure travelers, customizing them based on specific travel needs. Specialty kits are available for travelers managing diabetes, dealing with dental emergencies, and participating in aquatic activities. Many pharmacy, grocery, retail, and outdoor sporting goods stores, as well as online retailers, sell basic first aid kits. Travelers who choose to purchase a preassembled kit should review the contents carefully to ensure that it has everything needed; any necessary additional items should be added.[1]

---

[1] "Travel Health Kits," Centers for Disease Control and Prevention (CDC), May 1, 2023. Available online. URL: wwwnc.cdc.gov/travel/yellowbook/2024/preparing/travel-health-kits. Accessed July 31, 2024.

Part 6 | **Travelers with Special Needs**

Chapter 33 | **Health and Safety for Women Travelers**

In some places, women travelers may face extra health and security risks. Before you go, read these tips to help ensure a safe and healthy journey.

RESEARCH YOUR DESTINATION: BE AWARE OF LOCAL CUSTOMS AND NORMS

Customs and norms in other countries can differ greatly from those in the United States. Some countries have rules against certain behaviors or speech, while others have specific expectations regarding women's clothing and appearance. For example, tight-fitting clothes, sleeveless shirts, or shorts may not be acceptable.

WOMEN'S HEALTH ABROAD

Every country has its own health-care system. When traveling, bring health items that might be hard to find at your destination, such as feminine hygiene products or birth control. Many countries have laws that affect women's health differently than where you live. For instance, some countries make certain reproductive health services illegal. Others may punish women who become pregnant out of wedlock, including victims of sexual assault.

If you are pregnant, be aware that airlines might not let you fly in the later stages of pregnancy. It is advisable to have a note from your doctor stating that it is safe for you to fly. Additionally, ensure your travel insurance covers pregnancy-related costs.

PUBLIC TRANSPORT

The safety of public transportation varies widely from country to country. In many places, informal taxis or minibuses can be particularly dangerous for women traveling alone. To stay safe, consider the following transport tips:

- **Arrange transport to and from the airport before you arrive, using a licensed and reputable company**. This ensures you have a reliable and safe option waiting for you upon arrival, reducing the risk of falling prey to unlicensed or potentially dangerous drivers.
- **Do not hitchhike**. Hitchhiking poses significant safety risks as it involves getting into a vehicle with a stranger without any official record of the ride or the driver, increasing vulnerability to potential harm.
- **Research taxi and other ride-share companies before you go to ensure they are licensed and reputable**. This is crucial for your safety and can help you avoid unregulated or unsafe services.
- **Consider using app-based transportation companies**. These companies offer a record of your ride, unlike hailing a ride on the street. Some companies also allow a rider to share their real-time ride details with another person. This feature can help identify the vehicle and driver later.
- **Avoid traveling in busy sections of train cars or on crowded buses**. Public transportation can create opportunities for inappropriate or unwanted physical contact and facilitate pickpocketing.

TRAVEL ACCOMMODATIONS

When registering at lodging, use your first initial and avoid using titles such as "Mrs., Ms., or Miss." Additionally, do not disclose where you are staying to strangers. For more information, review the lodging safety guidelines (https://travel.state.gov/content/travel/en/international-travel/before-you-go/lodging-safety.html).

BE AWARE OF YOUR SURROUNDINGS

Use your best judgment to avoid unsafe situations. Plan ahead and develop a safety strategy for dealing with potential dangers. Consider bringing personal safety whistles or alarms and taking self-defense courses before your trip. In an unsafe situation, speaking loudly and drawing attention to yourself can deter unwanted actions. Remember, being safe is more important than being polite. Use facial expressions, body language, and a firm voice to avoid unwanted attention. Locate nearby emergency services, such as police stations and hospitals, in case of an emergency.

GENDER-BASED VIOLENCE

Gender-based violence (GBV) includes violence committed against someone because of their gender and disproportionately affects women and minorities worldwide. Forms of GBV include sexual or physical assault, domestic violence, forced marriage, female infanticide, sex and human trafficking, and other violent acts. Women travelers can be targeted for these crimes. If you are a victim of GBV, contact the Office of Overseas Citizens Services at 888-407-4747. If you are overseas, call 202-501-4444. You can also contact the nearest U.S. Embassy or Consulate (www.usembassy.gov).

DRUG-ASSISTED RAPE OR "DATE RAPE"

Drug-assisted rape, also known as "date rape," occurs when someone drugs another person to sexually assault them. The drugs are typically added to the victim's drink without their knowledge. Victims usually cannot detect the presence of drugs such as Rohypnol, ketamine, or scopolamine, which can render a person unconscious and defenseless. To protect yourself:

- Always watch your drink and cover it with your hand if possible.
- Do not accept drinks from strangers.
- Be aware of how much you are drinking and notice any unusual physical symptoms beyond normal intoxication.

- If you feel strange or sick, inform a trusted friend if possible and contact emergency authorities immediately. You can call local police or the nearest U.S. Embassy or Consulate.

If you are sexually assaulted or raped, seek medical care and resources. The nearest U.S. Embassy or Consulate can provide information on getting help and medical care in the country you are in, including whether postexposure prophylaxis (PEP) is available. It is crucial to receive medical care within 72 hours to prevent human immunodeficiency virus (HIV) and obtain emergency contraception. The Rape, Abuse, and Incest National Network (RAINN) is a U.S.-based organization that provides resources (www.rainn.org/resources) to sexual assault and abuse victims. They can offer support remotely or when you return to the United States.[1]

---

[1] Bureau of Consular Affairs, "Women Travelers," U.S. Department of State (DOS), February 28, 2024. Available online. URL: https://travel.state.gov/content/travel/en/international-travel/before-you-go/travelers-with-special-considerations/women-travelers.html. Accessed July 31, 2024.

Chapter 34 | **Safety Tips for Pregnant Travelers**

Pregnant travelers can generally travel safely with appropriate preparation, but they should avoid destinations with risks such as Zika and malaria. Here are some important considerations for safe travel during pregnancy.

BEFORE TRAVEL

- **Check airline and cruise policies.** Before booking a cruise or air travel, review the policies of the airlines or cruise operators regarding pregnant women. Some airlines allow travel up to 36 weeks, while others may have earlier cutoffs. Cruises may restrict travel after 24–28 weeks of pregnancy and may require a note from your doctor stating that you are fit to travel.
- **Consult with a health-care provider.** Schedule an appointment with your health-care provider or a travel health specialist (wwwnc.cdc.gov/travel/page/find-clinic) at least one month before departure. They can provide destination-specific vaccines, medicines, and information. Discussing your health concerns, itinerary, and planned activities with your provider allows them to give tailored advice and recommendations.
- **Plan for the unexpected.** It is essential to prepare for unexpected events to ensure access to quality health care and avoid being stranded. Take steps such as getting travel insurance (wwwnc.cdc.gov/travel/page/insurance), learning where to obtain health care during travel (wwwnc.cdc.gov/travel/page/health-care-during-travel),

packing a travel health kit, and enrolling in the U.S. Department of State's Smart Traveler Enrollment Program (STEP; https://step.state.gov/step). Ensure your health-care policy covers pregnancy and neonatal complications abroad. If not, consider purchasing travel health insurance that includes these items and medical evacuation insurance.

- **Recognize emergency signs**. Be aware of signs and symptoms that require immediate medical attention, including pelvic or abdominal pain, bleeding, contractions, symptoms of preeclampsia (unusual swelling, severe headaches, nausea and vomiting, and vision changes), and dehydration.
- **Prepare a travel health kit (wwwnc.cdc.gov/travel/page/pack-smart)**. Pregnant travelers should include prescription medications, hemorrhoid cream, antiemetic drugs, antacids, prenatal vitamins, medication for vaginitis or yeast infections, and support hose in addition to the items recommended for all travelers.

DURING TRAVEL

- **Prevent swelling and blood clots**. To avoid swelling and reduce the risk of blood clots or deep vein thrombosis (DVT), wear comfortable shoes and loose clothing. Try to walk around every hour or so during long flights. Your doctor may also recommend compression stockings or leg exercises to perform in your seat.
- **Choose safe food and drink**. Contaminated food or drinks can lead to travelers' diarrhea and other diseases, especially in low- or middle-income destinations (wwwnc.cdc.gov/travel/destinations/list). Generally, foods served hot, dry, and packaged foods are safe. Bottled, canned, and hot drinks are also usually safe. Pregnant women should avoid using bismuth subsalicylate, found in Pepto-Bismol and Kaopectate. Additionally, iodine tablets for water purification should not be used, as they can harm the thyroid development of the fetus.

Safety Tips for Pregnant Travelers

Traveling during pregnancy requires careful planning and consideration of potential risks. By consulting with health-care professionals, preparing appropriately, and being mindful of health and safety precautions, pregnant travelers can enjoy a safe and healthy journey. Always prioritize your well-being and seek medical advice when needed.[1]

[1] "Pregnant Travelers," Centers for Disease Control and Prevention (CDC), June 28, 2022. Available online. URL: wwwnc.cdc.gov/travel/page/pregnant-travelers. Accessed July 31, 2024.

Chapter 35 | **Traveling with Children**

HEALTH RISKS AND CONSIDERATIONS

Children may face the same health risks as their parents during travel, but the health consequences can be more serious. Some illnesses can be difficult to recognize in children, especially if they cannot yet express what they are feeling. Additionally, children may be more likely to encounter health risks, such as animals, due to their size and curiosity. If you plan to travel with children, familiarize yourself with the information on this page to help everyone stay safe and healthy.

PREDEPARTURE PREPARATIONS
Medical Consultation and Vaccinations
MAKE AN APPOINTMENT

Schedule a visit with your child's primary health-care professional or a travel medicine specialist at least one month before departure. They can provide destination-specific vaccines, medicines, and information. Discussing your itinerary and planned activities with your provider allows them to offer specific advice and recommendations.

ENSURE ROUTINE VACCINATIONS

Ensure your child is up-to-date on all routine vaccines. Routine vaccinations protect against infectious diseases, such as measles, which can spread quickly among unvaccinated groups. While many of these diseases are uncommon in the United States, they are still prevalent in other countries.

SPECIAL CONSIDERATIONS FOR ROUTINE VACCINES

Some routine vaccines for young children may have different recommendations for international travel. For example, while the first dose of the measles, mumps, rubella (MMR) vaccine is usually given after 12 months, infants aged 6–11 months should receive one dose before international travel. Some travel vaccines can be administered on an accelerated schedule, meaning doses are given in a shorter time frame. Not all travel vaccines can be administered to very young children, so consult a travel medicine doctor or your child's pediatrician early.

Planning for Unexpected Events

TRAVEL INSURANCE

It is important to prepare for unexpected events by obtaining travel insurance (wwwnc.cdc.gov/travel/page/insurance). Ensure you have medical and emergency evacuation insurance for your trip. Consider purchasing supplemental insurance, as U.S. Medicare and Medicaid do not cover medical costs overseas.

HEALTH-CARE ACCESS AND TRAVEL HEALTH KIT

Learn where to access health care during travel (wwwnc.cdc.gov/travel/page/health-care-during-travel) and pack a travel health kit (wwwnc.cdc.gov/travel/page/pack-smart). This includes obtaining travel insurance, knowing the location of nearby health-care facilities, and enrolling in the U.S. Department of State's Smart Traveler Enrollment Program (STEP; https://step.state.gov/step).

SMART TRAVELER ENROLLMENT PROGRAM

Enroll in STEP to receive important safety and security information. For travel updates, follow @TravelGov on Twitter, Facebook, and Instagram.[1]

---

[1] "Traveling with Children," Centers for Disease Control and Prevention (CDC), August 16, 2022. Available online. URL: wwwnc.cdc.gov/travel/page/children. Accessed July 31, 2024.

AIR TRAVEL IN-TRANSIT CONSIDERATIONS

While air travel is generally safe for most newborns, infants, and children, consider a few issues before departure. Children with chronic heart or lung conditions may be at risk for hypoxia during flights, so consult a clinician beforehand.

Ear Pain Management

Ear pain during descent can be troublesome for infants and children. Swallowing or chewing can help equalize pressure in the middle ear. Infants should nurse or suck on a bottle, and older children can try chewing gum. Antihistamines and decongestants are generally ineffective. Air travel does not exacerbate symptoms or complications associated with otitis media.

Jet Lag Management

Traveling across time zones can disrupt sleep patterns in children, similar to adults. Plan for rest and adjustments in the schedule accordingly.

Safety Restraints

Ensure children are safely restrained during flights. Severe turbulence or a crash can create enough momentum that an adult cannot hold onto a child. The safest place for a child on an airplane is in a government-approved child safety restraint system (CRS) or device. The Federal Aviation Administration (FAA) strongly recommends securing children in a CRS for the flight duration. Car seats cannot be used in all seats or planes, so check with the airline for specific restrictions and approved child restraint options.[2]

HEALTH CONCERNS DURING TRAVEL
Diarrhea

Diarrhea is a common illness among children traveling abroad and can lead to dehydration. The best treatment for children with

---

[2] "Traveling Safely with Infants and Children," Centers for Disease Control and Prevention (CDC), May 1, 2023. Available online. URL: wwwnc.cdc.gov/travel/yellowbook/2024/family/infants-and-children. Accessed July 31, 2024.

diarrhea is plenty of fluids; medication is usually unnecessary. If your child appears dehydrated, has a fever, or exhibits bloody stools, seek medical attention immediately. Consider the following:

- Oral rehydration salts (available online or in most developing countries) can prevent dehydration.
- Over-the-counter (OTC) drugs containing bismuth (Pepto-Bismol or Kaopectate) should not be used in children.
- Antibiotics are generally reserved for severe cases.
- Other treatments for diarrhea, such as loperamide, are not recommended for children under six years old.

Breastfeeding is the best way to prevent and manage diarrhea in infants. If using formula, bring your own supply and prepare it according to the manufacturer's instructions. If water quality is poor, use sterile water to prepare formula and sterilize bottles, nipples, caps, and rings. Sterilization can be done using a dishwasher, boiling in water for five minutes, a microwave steam sterilizer bag, or bleach if no other options are available.

Everyone should choose safer food and drinks to prevent diarrhea. Eat foods served hot, dry, or packaged. Drink bottled, canned, or hot beverages and only consume pasteurized milk. For short trips, consider bringing snacks from home when safe food is unavailable.

Wash hands with soap and water. If unavailable, use an alcohol-based hand sanitizer with at least 60 percent alcohol. Use soap and clean water to wash bottles, pacifiers, and toys that fall on the floor.

Diseases Spread by Bugs

Mosquitoes can transmit diseases such as Zika, chikungunya, malaria, dengue, and yellow fever. Ticks can spread diseases such as Lyme disease and tick-borne encephalitis.

Children can be protected from these diseases by using Environmental Protection Agency (EPA)-registered insect repellents (www.epa.gov/insect-repellents) containing active ingredients such as N,N-diethyl-meta-toluamide (DEET), picaridin, IR3535, oil of lemon eucalyptus (OLE), para-menthane-diol (PMD), or

2-undecanone. When using insect repellent on children, follow the label instructions. Spray repellent onto your hands before applying it to a child's face, and avoid using OLE or PMD on children under three years old. Do not apply repellent to a child's hands, eyes, mouth, cuts, or irritated skin. If also using sunscreen, apply it first.

Additional protective measures include dressing children in clothing that covers the arms and legs and covering strollers and baby carriers with mosquito netting.

Malaria

Malaria is a serious infection that children can contract while traveling internationally. Children visiting friends and relatives in areas with malaria may be at higher risk due to longer stays. Children traveling to malaria-endemic areas should take preventive medication. A health-care professional can recommend the appropriate medicine, and a pharmacist can prepare the medication in a child-friendly format if necessary. Malaria medications should be stored in childproof containers and kept out of reach of children. Even when taking malaria medication, use insect repellent and other measures to avoid bug bites.

Rabies

Rabies is primarily spread through contact with mammals. It is almost always fatal if not treated promptly. Children are at higher risk due to their size and tendency to play with animals. Supervise children around animals, especially dogs, puppies, cats, kittens, and wildlife. Any animal bite should be thoroughly washed with soap and water, and medical attention should be sought immediately.

SAFETY AND SECURITY
Road Safety

Children should always wear a seat belt or sit in appropriate car and booster seats. Research car seat guidelines for the destination country, as U.S. car seats may not be approved for use elsewhere. Generally, children are safest in the back seat. No one should travel in the back of a pickup truck. See Traffic and Road Safety (www. cdc.gov) for more tips.

Water Activities

Supervise children closely during water activities and ensure they wear a life jacket.[3]

Identification and Documentation

If family members become separated, each child should carry identifying information and contact numbers. Due to concerns about illegal child transport across international borders, parents traveling alone with children should carry relevant custody papers or a notarized permission letter from the other parent.

ADDITIONAL CONSIDERATIONS
Drinking Water Contaminants

Drinking water disinfection does not remove environmental contaminants such as lead or other metals. Travelers may want to carry specific filters designed to remove these contaminants, particularly when large amounts of water are consumed (e.g., long-term travel or living abroad).

Altitude Illness and Acute Mountain Sickness

Children are as susceptible to high-altitude effects as adults. A slow ascent is preferable to avoid acute mountain sickness (AMS). Young children may show nonspecific symptoms such as loss of appetite or irritability, while older children might report headaches or shortness of breath. If unexplained symptoms occur after an ascent, a descent may be necessary.

Insurance

Before departure, verify insurance coverage for illnesses and injuries abroad. Consider purchasing special medical evacuation insurance (wwwnc.cdc.gov/travel/yellowbook/2024/health-care-abroad/insurance) for airlift or air ambulance transport to facilities that provide adequate medical care.

---

[3] See footnote [1].

Travel Stress

Changes in schedule, activities, and environment can be stressful for children. To reduce stress, involve children in planning and bring familiar toys or objects. For children with chronic illnesses, consult with health-care providers about timing and itinerary decisions.[4]

---

[4] See footnote [2].

Chapter 36 | **Travel Safety Tips for Older Adults**

If you are an older adult considering international travel, you must take specific precautions to ensure a safe and healthy trip. Here are some tips and guidelines to help you prepare.

BEFORE YOU TRAVEL

- **Check the Centers for Disease Control and Prevention's (CDC) travel website**. Visit the CDC web page (wwwnc. cdc.gov/travel/destinations/list) for your destination to find out which vaccines or medicines you may need and what diseases or health risks exist.
- **Schedule a health consultation**. Make an appointment with your health-care provider or a travel health specialist (wwwnc.cdc.gov/travel/page/find-clinic) at least one month before departure. They can provide destination-specific vaccines, medicines, and information. Discussing your health concerns, itinerary, and planned activities with your provider allows them to offer specific advice and recommendations.
- **Inform your doctor about**:
  - any chronic medical conditions, such as hypertension and asthma
  - all destinations you will visit
  - types of accommodations, such as hotels, hostels, short-term rentals, boats, camping, and so on.
  - the purpose of your trip, such as visiting friends and relatives (VFR), business, or adventure travel
  - the timing and length of your trip

- planned activities, such as climbing at high altitudes, scuba diving, humanitarian aid work, or taking cruises
- all medications you are taking
- **Update routine vaccinations**. Ensure you are up-to-date on all routine vaccines, including the pneumococcal pneumonia vaccine, zoster or shingles vaccine, and an annual flu shot. Routine vaccinations protect against infectious diseases, such as measles, which can spread quickly in unvaccinated groups. While many of these diseases are rare in the United States, they are still common in other countries.
- **Take recommended medicines as directed**. If your doctor prescribes medicine, take it as directed before, during, and after travel. Counterfeit drugs are common in some countries, so only take medication you bring from home. Pack enough for your trip and extra in case of delays.
- **Keep a medical record**. Carry a paper or electronic record of your medical history during travel.

CRUISE SHIP TRAVEL

Cruises are popular among older adults but can create ideal conditions for spreading diseases like norovirus and respiratory illnesses such as influenza and coronavirus 2019 (COVID-19). To reduce your risk:

- Wash your hands frequently, especially before eating and after using the bathroom.
- Avoid touching your face with unwashed hands.
- Reschedule your trip if you feel sick before departure. If you feel unwell during the voyage, report your symptoms to the ship's medical facility and follow their recommendations.

PLAN FOR THE UNEXPECTED

- **Get travel insurance (wwwnc.cdc.gov/travel/page/insurance)**. Determine if your health insurance covers medical care abroad (wwwnc.cdc.gov/travel/page/getting-health-care-abroad). Travelers are usually responsible for paying hospital and medical expenses out-of-pocket in most destinations. Consider purchasing additional insurance that covers health care and emergency evacuation, especially if traveling to remote areas. There are various types of travel insurance, including trip cancellation insurance, travel health insurance, and medical evacuation insurance.

- **Enroll in Smart Traveler Enrollment Program (STEP).** Register with the U.S. Department of State's STEP (https://step.state.gov/step) to receive updates on Travel Advisories and ensure that the DOS can contact you in case of serious legal, medical, or financial issues. In an emergency at home, STEP can also help friends and family reach you.
- **Learn basic first aid and cardiopulmonary resuscitation (CPR).** These skills can be invaluable. Bring a travel health kit (wwwnc.cdc.gov/travel/page/pack-smart) and familiarize yourself with emergency services numbers at your destination.

AFTER TRAVEL

- **Monitor your health**. If you feel sick after traveling, especially with a fever, talk to a health-care provider. Be sure to inform them about any areas you recently traveled to, as this information can be crucial for diagnosing and treating potential illnesses.
- **Seek medical care abroad**. For more information on accessing health care while traveling, see the Getting Health Care During Travel page (www.cdc.gov/travel/page/getting-health-care-during-travel).

Traveling as an older adult requires careful planning and awareness of potential health and safety issues. By consulting health-care professionals, updating vaccinations, and preparing for unexpected events, you can enjoy a safe and fulfilling journey.[1]

---

[1] "Older Adults and Healthy Travel," Centers for Disease Control and Prevention (CDC), January 31, 2022. Available online. URL: wwwnc.cdc.gov/travel/page/senior-citizens. Accessed July 31, 2024.

Chapter 37 | **Safety Tips for LGBTQI+ Travelers**

Lesbian, gay, bisexual, transgender, queer, and intersex (LGBTQI+) travelers may encounter special challenges while traveling abroad. Laws and attitudes vary significantly from country to country, affecting the safety and ease of travel. About 70 countries criminalize consensual same-sex relations, and some countries do not recognize same-sex marriage. In certain regions, engaging in same-sex sexual relations can lead to severe punishment. Here are some essential tips and considerations for LGBTQI+ travelers.

BEFORE YOU TRAVEL
Research Your Destination
Review the country information page (https://travel.state.gov/content/travel/en/international-travel/International-Travel-Country-Information-Pages.html) for your destination. These pages provide specific information for LGBTQI+ travelers, including legal considerations and cultural attitudes.

Information for Travelers with an X Gender Marker on Their Passport
U.S. citizens can select an X as their gender marker on their U.S. passport application. For information on X gender marker passports and the process for changing your gender marker, visit the Selecting Your Gender Marker page (https://travel.state.gov/content/travel/en/passports/need-passport/selecting-your-gender-marker.html). While the U.S. government issues passports with the X gender marker, it cannot guarantee entry or transit through other countries, as some may not recognize this marker.

Check with the foreign embassy or consulate in the United States before traveling.

Pack Important Documents

Bring copies of essential documents, especially in countries with different laws from the United States. These documents may include:

- legal and health documents, such as a living will or health-care directive
- parentage and/or custody documents for accompanying minor children, particularly if they do not share your last name or if only one parent is traveling with the children
- contact information for your family and/or attorney in the United States, including someone with a copy of your itinerary
- address and phone number of the nearest U.S. Embassy or Consulate (www.usembassy.gov), in both English and the local language

Consider Buying Insurance

Travel insurance can be crucial during emergencies, including medical evacuation. Some insurance products are specifically designed for LGBTQI+ travelers. Ensure that any insurance you purchase covers all family members traveling with you.

Enroll in the Smart Traveler Enrollment Program

The Smart Traveler Enrollment Program (STEP; https://step.state.gov/step) is a free service for U.S. citizens traveling to or living in a foreign country. The U.S. Department of State (DOS) encourages all travelers to enroll in STEP. By entering information about your upcoming trip, the DOS can send you current Travel Advisories and Alerts. Include an email address or phone number to be reached in an emergency.

Note: *The X gender marker option is not yet available in STEP due to the technological updates needed. However, gender is not a required field on the enrollment form. The DOS is working on updating systems to include the X gender marker.*

WHILE YOU ARE THERE

- **Be aware of local laws**. You are subject to the laws of the country you visit (https://travel.state.gov/content/travel/en/international-travel/International-Travel-Country-Information-Pages.html). In some places, same-sex marriage and consensual same-sex relations are illegal. Public gatherings supporting LGBTQI+ communities or sharing pro-LGBTQI+ material may also be banned.
- **Watch for entrapment campaigns**. Police in some countries monitor websites, apps, and meeting places. Be cautious when connecting with locals.
- **Be cautious with new acquaintances**. Criminals may target or attempt to extort foreigners perceived to be LGBTQI+.
- **Know the local attitudes**. Some resorts or neighborhoods may be welcoming, but nearby areas might be less accepting. Be cautious when planning excursions outside the resort or area.

LIVING ABROAD WITH YOUR FOREIGN NATIONAL SPOUSE OR PARTNER

Check the foreign embassy or consulate website (www.state.gov/resources-for-foreign-embassies/diplomatic-list) to learn whether same-sex relationships are legal and if special documentation, such as work authorization or a residence visa, is required.

IF YOU NEED HELP, CONTACT THE U.S. EMBASSY OR CONSULATE

If you encounter problems overseas, especially if you feel unsafe approaching local police or have had issues with them, the nearest U.S. Embassy or Consulate can assist you.

- Consular officers will protect your privacy and will not make assumptions or judgments.
- Report any poor treatment or harassment to them.
- If arrested, immediately request the police to notify the U.S. Embassy.

Traveling as an LGBTQI+ individual requires careful preparation and awareness of local laws and cultural attitudes. By staying informed and taking necessary precautions, you can help ensure a safer and more enjoyable trip.[1]

---

[1] Bureau of Consular Affairs, "LGBTQI+ Travelers," U.S. Department of State (DOS), March 11, 2024. Available online. URL: https://travel.state.gov/content/travel/en/international-travel/before-you-go/travelers-with-special-considerations/lgbtqi.html. Accessed July 31, 2024.

Chapter 38 | Travel Guidelines for Immunocompromised Individuals

Immunocompromised individuals, including organ transplant recipients and those with various other conditions, often face unique health challenges and increased risks when traveling. Careful pretravel preparation and consideration of specific medical needs are crucial for ensuring their safety and well-being during international travel.

APPROACH TO IMMUNIZATIONS
When preparing immunocompromised travelers for international travel, it is essential to consider their medical history and underlying conditions. Not all medical conditions require special considerations for pretravel immunizations, but all appropriate travel vaccines should be recommended and provided. This can help protect travelers from vaccine-preventable diseases they may encounter abroad.

VACCINE CONSIDERATIONS FOR TRAVELERS WITH SEVERE IMMUNE COMPROMISE
Severely immunocompromised individuals include those with conditions such as aplastic anemia, graft-versus-host disease, symptomatic HIV/AIDS, certain congenital immunodeficiencies,

active leukemia or lymphoma, and generalized malignancy. Others with severe immune compromise include individuals who have recently received radiation therapy or checkpoint inhibitor treatment, those receiving active immunosuppression for solid organ transplants, and both chimeric antigen receptor (CAR)-T cell and hematopoietic stem cell transplant (HSCT) recipients within two years of transplantation or while still taking immunosuppressive drugs.

In most cases, severely immunocompromised individuals should avoid live vaccines, which can pose significant risks. Inactivated vaccines are safer but may be less effective due to the suppressed immune response. It is often advisable for these individuals to postpone travel until their immune function improves. For those who may travel in the future, initiating travel-related vaccines before starting immunosuppressive therapies can be beneficial. Whenever possible, inactivated vaccines should be administered at least two weeks before immunosuppression begins, and live vaccines should be given at least four weeks prior.

ORGAN TRANSPLANT RECIPIENTS

Specific considerations are necessary when prescribing travel-related medications for organ transplant recipients. Atovaquone-proguanil is often the most appropriate malaria prophylactic agent because it is less likely to interact with calcineurin inhibitors and mTor inhibitors (cyclosporine, everolimus, sirolimus, tacrolimus). Other antimalarials, such as chloroquine, doxycycline, mefloquine, and primaquine, can elevate calcineurin inhibitor levels and may prolong the QT interval when used in conjunction with these inhibitors. Additionally, some travel-related medications may require dose adjustments based on altered hepatic or renal function.

DEVELOPING A PLAN IN CASE OF ILLNESS
- **Identifying appropriate health-care facilities**.
  It is important to locate clinics or hospitals in the destination country capable of providing care to immunocompromised patients.

- **Accessing U.S. Embassy resources**. It is vital to understand how to access and utilize embassy resources in an emergency.
- **Securing supplemental insurance**. It is recommended that you purchase insurance to cover trip cancellation due to illness, health-care costs abroad, and medical evacuation.

FOOD AND WATER PRECAUTIONS

- **Adhering to safe food and water guidelines**. To minimize the risk of foodborne illnesses, following strict precautions is essential.
- **Safe hygiene practices**. Utilizing antibacterial hand wipes or an alcohol-based hand sanitizer containing at least 60 percent alcohol is advisable.

MULTIDRUG-RESISTANT ORGANISMS

Immunocompromised individuals are at a heightened risk of infection with multidrug-resistant organisms. It is important to notify health-care providers about any posttravel illness and provide comprehensive travel details.

MEDICATIONS

- **Carrying extra medications**. It is advisable to bring extra supplies of medications to account for potential travel delays, ensuring all medications are labeled and kept in their original packaging.
- **Avoiding locally purchased medications**. Medications bought at the destination may pose risks due to possible drug-drug interactions and the potential presence of counterfeit, falsely labeled, falsified, spurious, or substandard products.

SUN PROTECTION

- **Increased risk of skin cancer**. Immunocompromised individuals have a significantly higher risk of developing skin cancer.

- **Preventing photosensitivity**. Some medications can increase photosensitivity; therefore, it is crucial to use sun protection, including sunscreen, protective clothing, and hats.

OBTAINING HEALTH CARE ABROAD

Travelers might seek medical care abroad for various issues, from self-limited minor ailments to chronic conditions or major illnesses and injuries. It is essential to understand that insurance plans may not cover emergency health care abroad. Travelers should check with their insurance carriers before departure to confirm the limits of their coverage and identify any additional coverage requirements. For instance, travel health insurance alone often does not cover the cost of emergency medical evacuation or itinerary changes needed to receive medical care. Specific policies can be purchased to cover these expenses, but they may not include costs related to preexisting conditions.

TRAVEL HEALTH KIT SUPPLIES

It is essential to provide detailed instructions and information about any prescribed medications, including antibiotics for self-treatment of diarrhea, medications for altitude illness, and malaria chemoprophylaxis.

Understanding the unique risks and taking appropriate measures can help ensure a safer and more comfortable journey. Consulting with health-care professionals for personalized advice and support before traveling is highly recommended.[1]

---

[1] "Immunocompromised Travelers," Centers for Disease Control and Prevention (CDC), May 1, 2023. Available online. URL: wwwnc.cdc.gov/travel/yellowbook/2024/additional-considerations/immunocompromised-travelers. Accessed July 31, 2024.

Chapter 39 | **Travelers with Chronic Illnesses**

Traveling abroad can be relaxing, but the physical demands of travel can be challenging, especially for travelers with chronic illnesses such as heart disease, diabetes, asthma, or arthritis. Proper planning and preparation can help ensure a safe and comfortable trip.

BEFORE TRAVEL

- **Make an appointment**. Schedule a visit with your health-care provider or a travel health specialist (wwwnc. cdc.gov/travel/page/find-clinic) at least one month before departure. They can provide destination-specific vaccines, medicines, and information. Discussing your health concerns, itinerary, and planned activities with your provider allows them to give specific advice and recommendations.
- **Check the Centers for Disease Control and Prevention's (CDC) website**. Visit the CDC's web page (wwwnc. cdc.gov/travel/destinations/list) for your destination to determine which vaccines or medicines you may need and what diseases or health risks are present there.
- **Take recommended medicines as directed**. If your doctor prescribes medication, take it as directed before, during, and after travel. Counterfeit drugs are common in some countries, so only take medication you bring from home. Ensure you pack enough for the duration of your trip, plus extra in case of travel delays.
- **Prevent drug interactions**. Inform your health-care provider about all the medications you routinely take

before they prescribe any new medications for travel. Some vaccines cannot be given to individuals taking certain medications, and some medicines, such as steroids, can weaken the immune system, making you more susceptible to travel-related infections.

- **Manage medication supplies.** Insurance companies may cover only a 30-day supply of medications at a time. If your trip extends beyond this period, discuss with your health-care provider and insurance company how to obtain enough medicine for the entire duration of your trip.
- **Check medication restrictions.** Verify with the U.S. Embassy or Consulate (www.usembassy.gov) if there are any restrictions on bringing specific medications into your destination country.
- **Notify your airline.** If you require oxygen or other medical equipment, inform your airline well in advance. The Transportation Security Administration (TSA) Cares Helpline (toll-free at 855-787-2227) can provide information on preparing for airport security screening with respect to particular disabilities or medical conditions.
- **Get travel insurance.** Determine if your health insurance covers medical care abroad. Travelers are typically responsible for paying hospital and other medical expenses out-of-pocket at most destinations. Ensure you have a plan for receiving care overseas. Consider purchasing additional insurance that covers health care and emergency evacuation, especially if traveling to remote areas.
- **Plan for the unexpected.** Preparing for unexpected events can help you access quality health care or avoid being stranded at a destination. Steps to consider include:
  - obtaining travel insurance (wwwnc.cdc.gov/travel/page/insurance)
  - learning where to access health care during travel (wwwnc.cdc.gov/travel/page/health-care-during-travel)
  - packing a travel health kit (wwwnc.cdc.gov/travel/page/pack-smart)

- enrolling in the U.S. Department of State's (DOS) Smart Traveler Enrollment Program (STEP; https://step.state.gov/step)

DURING TRAVEL

- **Carry a health information card**. Include details about your health conditions and a list of your medications, written in English and, if possible, the local language. Consider bringing copies of x-rays or other imaging, recent lab results, your most recent electrocardiogram (ECG or EKG), and other relevant medical documentation. Wearing a medical alert bracelet or other medical jewelry with this information is advisable if appropriate.
- **Maintain healthy habits**. Practice healthy habits, such as eating nutritious food and exercising regularly. Continue taking recommended medicines as directed.
- **Prevent blood clots**. Airplane travel, especially flights longer than four hours, may increase the risk of blood clots, including deep vein thrombosis (DVT) and pulmonary embolism (PE). Certain chronic diseases also elevate this risk. Select an aisle seat when possible to allow for walking every two to three hours to help prevent blood clots.

Note: *The U.S. Embassy at your destination can help you locate medical services and notify family and friends in an emergency.*

AFTER TRAVEL

If you have traveled and feel unwell, especially if you develop a fever, consult a health-care provider as soon as possible. It is important to inform them about any regions you recently visited, as this information can assist in diagnosing and treating potential travel-related illnesses.[1]

---

[1] "Travelers with Chronic Illnesses," Centers for Disease Control and Prevention (CDC), August 16, 2022. Available online. URL: wwwnc.cdc.gov/travel/page/chronic-illnesses. Accessed July 31, 2024.

Chapter 40 | Travel Planning for Individuals with Disabilities

Preparing for a trip is critical, especially for travelers with special considerations. Research and plan ahead to ensure a smooth and comfortable travel experience.

TRAVEL PREPARATIONS

- **Consult with travel service providers.** Contact your travel agent, hotel, airline, or cruise ship company to inquire about accessible accommodations and services during your trip and at your destination. Ask about rules for traveling with a service animal and any regulations for assistive devices on various modes of transport.
- **Transportation Security Administration (TSA) assistance.** Call the TSA's helpline at 855-787-2227 (toll-free) for help with the security screening process, procedures, and security checkpoints.
- **Overseas disability organizations.** Check websites such as Mobility International USA (www.miusa.org) to find overseas disability organizations.
- **The Hidden Disabilities Sunflower program.** This program, available in over 230 airports, helps travelers with hidden disabilities by allowing them to wear a Hidden Disabilities Sunflower lanyard or related aid. These items, available at participating airport information desks, signal to staff that the wearer may need assistance.

- **Human rights and social service framework.**
  For information about the rights of individuals
  with disabilities in your destination country,
  read Section 6 of the State Department's annual
  Human Rights Report (www.state.gov/reports-
  bureau-of-democracy-human-rights-and-labor/
  country-reports-on-human-rights-practices).
- **Airport help services.** Check the help services provided at
  your destination airport.

RESEARCH YOUR DESTINATION

Each country has its own laws regarding discrimination and
accessibility for persons with disabilities. Before traveling, visit
this website (https://travel.state.gov/destination) to find information for travelers with disabilities in the Local Laws and Special
Circumstances section. Be aware that in some countries, there may
be little to no requirement for accessibility, which can affect your
travel experience.

SERVICE ANIMALS

Research for traveling with a service animal:

- Before traveling, check the Country Information Page
  (https://travel.state.gov/content/travel/en/international-
  travel/International-Travel-Country-Information-
  Pages.html) for information on legal limits, access
  issues, or cultural norms that may affect travel with
  your service animal.
- Investigate any quarantine, vaccination, or
  documentation requirements for your destination and
  any transit countries.
- Consult with your vet for tips on traveling with your
  service animal, and confirm with your hotel and airline
  that they will accommodate it.
- For more information, view Mobility International USA's
  tip sheet (www.miusa.org/resource/tip-sheets/disability-
  resources) for service dogs and international travel.

ASSISTIVE DEVICES AND EQUIPMENT

- **Airline rules**. Research airline policies regarding assistive devices and equipment, such as wheelchairs, portable machines, batteries, respirators, and oxygen. There may be specific rules for carrying these items as checked baggage or carry-ons. Security screening at both departing and arriving airports may also have specific regulations.
- **Medical equipment providers**. Investigate whether there are wheelchair and medical equipment providers at your destination and check for repair service availability. Considerations for wheelchairs and other assistive devices include:
  - rules about wheelchairs, including types (manual vs. power) and other devices like scooters
  - bringing extra supplies, such as wheelchair tires, tubes, and patch kits, as they may not be available at your destination
  - gate-checking your wheelchair and keeping the receipt
  - having information about your equipment, including make and model, and battery type, if any
  - checking airline policies on damaged equipment and replacement timelines
  - verifying the voltage of electricity at your destination and compatibility with your power wheelchair, which may require a converter
  - checking the type of electrical plug and outlets and bringing an adaptor if needed
  - considering the reliability of the electrical system at your destination
  - bringing extra batteries for devices such as hearing aids
  - carrying a portable external charger for equipment like communication devices

DEAF AND HARD-OF-HEARING TRAVELERS: VIDEO RELAY SERVICE

Deaf and hard-of-hearing travelers may choose to use a Video Relay Service (VRS) while overseas. To maintain access to VRS, travelers may need to register an account with their VRS provider before traveling and notify the provider before their trip. This ensures continued access to the service while abroad. There are several useful VRS websites that can be accessed while traveling, providing vital communication support.

MEDICAL CONSIDERATIONS

- **Consult with your physician**. Before traveling overseas, discuss your health-care needs with your doctor. U.S. Medicare/Medicaid does not provide coverage overseas, and private health insurance may not cover claims or require upfront payments before reimbursement. It is advisable to purchase supplemental medical insurance and medical evacuation plans.
- **Carry medical alert information**. Bring emergency contacts and a letter from your health-care provider detailing your medical condition, allergies, medications, potential complications, and other important information.
- **Manage prescription medications**. Carry sufficient prescription medication to last your entire trip, plus extra in case of delays. Note that some prescription medications legal in the United States may be illegal in other countries. Always carry prescriptions in their labeled containers, not in a pill pack, and pack medications in carry-on luggage. For medications requiring refrigeration, consider how to transport them, such as using an insulated bag, and request a hotel room with a small refrigerator. Bring extra supplies, such as incontinence supplies, diabetes test strips, and hearing aid batteries, which may not be available at your destination.
- **Locate medical services**. Research the type of medical services available at your destination, including hospitals, urgent care facilities, and dialysis centers.

COMMUNICATIONS

- **Stay informed**. Some airports may not have real-time alerts on screens. Sign up for alerts with your airline to receive up-to-date information, such as gate changes, delays, and cancellations. Check with your airline's service desk for assistance.

STAY CONNECTED

Enroll in the Smart Traveler Enrollment Program (STEP; https://step.state.gov) to receive security messages. STEP also makes it easier for the U.S. Embassy or Consulate to contact you in an emergency.[1]

---

[1] Bureau of Consular Affairs, "Travelers with Disabilities," U.S. Department of State (DOS), February 28, 2024. Available online. URL: https://travel.state.gov/content/travel/en/international-travel/before-you-go/travelers-with-special-considerations/traveling-with-disabilties.html. Accessed July 31, 2024.

Chapter 41 | Mental Health Considerations for International Travelers

International travel can be stressful, with the stress level varying depending on the type of travel. Short-term tourist travel is generally less stressful, while frequent travel, humanitarian and disaster work, and expatriation can be more challenging. Travel stress can trigger preexisting psychiatric disorders, reveal latent or undiagnosed issues, and lead to new mental health problems. Factors such as jet lag, fatigue, pandemics, and work or family pressures can contribute to anxiety and exacerbate depressive symptoms in short-term travelers.

OCCURRENCE OF MENTAL HEALTH PROBLEMS IN TRAVELERS

Data on the prevalence of mental health problems among travelers are limited. A study of British diplomats found that 11 percent of medical evacuations were for psychological reasons, with 71 percent of these individuals in their 20s. Depression accounted for 41 percent of these evacuations. In the U.S. Foreign Service from 1982 to 1986, psychiatric evacuations occurred at a rate of 0.2 percent, with 50 percent related to substance use or affective disorders. A study of psychiatric emergencies in travelers to Hawaii estimated rates of 0.2 percent for tourists, 2 percent for transient travelers, and 1 percent for residents. Diagnoses included schizophrenia, alcohol abuse, anxiety reactions, and depression. In a landscape analysis of travel-related psychosis, the estimated incidence of psychiatric hospitalization for tourists to Jerusalem was 19.7 cases per

100,000, with about 3.5 percent of these cases being psychotic episodes without a prior psychiatric history.

THE PRETRAVEL CONSULTATION AND MENTAL HEALTH EVALUATION

Travel health providers should include mental health screening in any pretravel consultation, especially for those planning extended or frequent travel, engaging in humanitarian or disaster relief work, or relocating long-term. While travel medicine specialists may not have mental health credentials, they should conduct a brief inquiry to identify any previously diagnosed psychiatric disorders. Providers can frame this inquiry by acknowledging that international travel is stressful and may trigger or exacerbate mental health issues.

Key areas to explore include past psychiatric disorders, any treatments received (inpatient, outpatient, or medications), current psychiatric conditions, family history of mental health issues, and current or past use of illicit substances. A history of inpatient treatment, psychotic episodes, violent or suicidal behavior, affective disorders, or substance use disorders warrants further evaluation by a mental health professional. Additionally, any abnormal mental status during the pretravel consultation should prompt a referral for further assessment.

CHALLENGES AND BARRIERS TO HEALTHY TRAVEL

Travelers with mental health issues may encounter several challenges and barriers, including:

- **Contraindicated medications**. Mefloquine can cause neuropsychiatric side effects and should be avoided for malaria prophylaxis in patients with mental health issues.
- **Laboratory monitoring of medication levels**. Travelers requiring routine laboratory testing for medications such as lithium should be informed of potential challenges in locating suitable facilities abroad. They should also be aware of the risk of lithium toxicity in high-temperature environments.

- **Medical evacuation insurance.** Travelers with mental health issues should consider purchasing international travel health and medical evacuation insurance (wwwnc.cdc.gov/travel/yellowbook/2024/health-care-abroad/insurance) that includes coverage for psychiatric emergencies. However, many policies exclude psychiatric emergencies or preexisting conditions.
- **Mental health treatment.** Long-term travelers or expatriates may have difficulty finding culturally compatible mental health treatment. They should seek guidance from a mental health professional with experience in international travel issues.
- **Refilling prescriptions.** Obtaining refills of psychotropic medications abroad may be challenging due to varying availability and legality. Travelers should consult the destination country's embassy or a reputable pharmacy or health-care provider.
- **Support groups.** Travelers with substance use disorders may seek support from organizations such as Alcoholics Anonymous (AA) or Narcotics Anonymous (NA). They should verify meeting availability and language in advance.
- **Traveling with psychotropic medications.** Customs regulations may prohibit certain medications (www.dea.gov/drug-information/drug-scheduling) used to treat mental health disorders. Travelers should carry medications in their original containers with a letter from the prescribing physician and check with the host country's embassy for restrictions.

STRESSORS AND COUNTERMEASURES

- **Culture shock.** Culture shock can result from the loss of familiar surroundings and routines, causing mood changes and adjustment difficulties. Foreknowledge and preparation can minimize its effect. Travelers should consider regular exercise, moderation in intoxicant use, adequate sleep and nutrition, and relaxation techniques to manage stress.

- **Jet lag**. A common, manageable stressor for most international travelers.
- **Travel during a pandemic**. The COVID-19 (coronavirus 2019) pandemic has heightened travel-related stress. Travelers should consider measures to control their personal health, mitigate COVID-19 risks, and plan for contingencies. They should consider travel health insurance covering cancellations and medical care related to COVID-19 and be prepared for different travel experiences due to pandemic restrictions.

POSTTRAVEL MENTAL HEALTH ISSUES

Travelers exposed to traumatic or life-threatening events may develop acute stress disorder (ASD) or posttraumatic stress disorder (PTSD). Humanitarian aid workers, disaster relief workers, and war correspondents are at higher risk. Clinicians should inquire about symptoms of ASD or PTSD and educate travelers about potential delayed reactions. Those experiencing symptoms should seek help from a mental health professional.

Mental health considerations are crucial for travelers, particularly those with preexisting conditions or exposure to high-stress situations. Proper screening, preparation, and support can help manage the challenges of international travel and mitigate the risk of mental health issues.[1]

---

[1] "Mental Health," Centers for Disease Control and Prevention (CDC), May 1, 2023. Available online. URL: wwwnc. cdc.gov/travel/yellowbook/2024/preparing/mental-health. Accessed July 31, 2024.

Chapter 42 | **Traveling with Pets and Service Animals**

TRAVELING WITH PETS

Taking your dog or cat on an international flight requires careful preparation. Ensure you have your pet's necessary documents when traveling abroad and returning to the United States. Start the process early to manage your pet's medical care and paperwork requirements.

First Stop—Your Vet's Office

If traveling internationally, inform your veterinarian about your plans as soon as possible. Together, you can ensure your pet is healthy enough to travel and meets the destination country's and the United States' requirements for return. Requirements may include:

- blood tests
- vaccinations
- microchips for identification
- permits
- health certificates

Airlines and countries often have different requirements, so be sure to verify the specific requirements for your destination.

Airlines

Different airlines have different rules regarding pet travel. Depending on the airline, your pet may be able to travel in the cabin or the cargo hold. Confirm your pet's travel arrangements with the airline ahead of time. Generally, only small dogs and cats that fit in special carriers under the seat are allowed in the cabin, where owners must care for them during layovers. Some airlines may not permit pets in the cabin, instead transporting them as cargo in a heated and ventilated hold. According to the International Air Transport Association, cats and dogs may travel and rest better in the cargo hold, as it is quieter and darker.

Pets can also travel as air cargo shipments on separate flights. If this is necessary due to your pet's size or destination country rules, acclimate your pet to the shipping kennel beforehand. Ensure the kennel door latches securely to prevent mishaps during transit. Consult your veterinarian for advice on feeding and watering. Arrangements for pickup at the final destination must be made for pets traveling as air cargo.

Some U.S. carriers do not allow pets to be shipped between May and September due to the heat. Regardless of the season, pets traveling as cargo must be in a sturdy container with adequate space to stand, sit, turn around, and lie down comfortably. Visit the U.S. Department of Agriculture's pet travel website (www.aphis.usda. gov/aphis/pet-travel) for more information. During connecting flights, care for pets traveling in the cabin, while airline staff or ground handlers care for those in cargo. Check with your airline(s) beforehand for specific requirements.

CONSIDER YOUR PET'S COMFORT
Loading and unloading can be stressful for pets. Consider these tips:
- Get your pet used to its carrier before the flight.
- Book flights with fewer connections or layovers.
- Choose departure and arrival times to avoid extreme temperatures, such as a nighttime arrival to a hot destination.
- Consult with your veterinarian. The International Air Transport Association discourages the use of sedatives or tranquilizers, as they could harm animals during flight.
- Walk your pet before leaving home and again before checking in.
- Check in as late as possible if your pet is allowed in the cabin to reduce stress.

- Check in early if your pet will be transported as cargo, allowing it to go to the quiet and dimly lit hold of the plane.

Cruise Ships and Travel by Sea

Different cruise lines have different rules about pets or service animals and required documents. Confirm these ahead of time with your cruise line. Pets traveling internationally on cruise ships or other maritime vessels must meet federal entry requirements to enter or reenter the United States. Note that the Centers for Disease Control and Prevention (CDC) has temporarily suspended the importation of dogs from countries considered high risk for dog rabies, including those that have visited such countries in the past six months.

Requirements for Dogs Leaving and Arriving in the United States

The CDC does not impose requirements for dogs leaving the United States. However, dogs returning to the United States must meet the same entry requirements as those from foreign countries. All dogs must appear healthy, and there is a temporary suspension for dogs imported from high-risk rabies countries. Some states may require vaccinations and health certificates, so check with your destination state's health department (www.aphis.usda.gov/aphis/pet-travel) before traveling. Certain breeds may face restrictions from airlines, cities, or states, so verify these before traveling.

The U.S. Department of Agriculture imposes additional restrictions on some dogs entering the United States, such as working dogs and those intended for resale or adoption.

Requirements for Cats Arriving in the United States

The CDC does not require a rabies vaccination certificate for cats entering the United States. However, many states and other countries do require it, and the CDC recommends rabies vaccination for all cats. Check the requirements for your destination and consult with your veterinarian before traveling.

Other Kinds of Pets

Different requirements may apply if your pet is not a cat or dog. Certain animals, such as primates (monkeys and apes) or African rodents, are not allowed back into the United States, even if they originated there.

Illness or Death of a Pet during Travel

Despite precautions, pets may become ill or die during a flight. Public health officials must ensure that the animal did not die from a communicable disease. They may perform an animal autopsy or other tests at your expense, and the animal's remains may not be returned after testing.

Consider Other Options

Ensure your pet is healthy enough for air travel. If there are doubts, consider leaving your pet with a trusted friend, family member, or boarding kennel or choosing another mode of transportation. Proper planning ensures that your pet arrives healthy and safe.[1]

SERVICE ANIMALS

Under the Air Carrier Access Act (ACAA), a service animal is a dog trained to perform tasks for an individual with a disability. Airlines must recognize and transport service dogs but are not required to transport other species or emotional support animals.

Things to Know
RECOGNITION AND TRANSPORT OF SERVICE ANIMALS

Airlines must recognize service dogs and accept them for transport on flights to, within, and from the United States. Although not required, airlines may transport other species at their discretion.

---

[1] "Traveling with Pets," Centers for Disease Control and Prevention (CDC), May 26, 2022. Available online. URL: www.cdc.gov/importation/traveling-with-pets.html. Accessed July 31, 2024.

CIRCUMSTANCES FOR DENYING TRANSPORT
Airlines may deny transport to a service dog if it:
- violates safety requirements, such as being too large or heavy
- poses a direct threat to others' health or safety
- causes significant disruption in the cabin or at airport gate areas
- violates health requirements, such as those prohibiting entry into a U.S. territory or foreign country

DETERMINING IF AN ANIMAL IS A SERVICE ANIMAL
Airlines may ask if the animal is required for a disability and what tasks it performs. They can look for physical indicators like a harness or vest and observe the animal's behavior.

REQUIRED DOCUMENTATION
Airlines may require a U.S. DOT form (www.transportation.gov/resources/individuals/aviation-consumer-protection/us-department-transportation-service-animal-air) attesting to the animal's health, behavior, and training, and another form (www.transportation.gov/resources/individuals/aviation-consumer-protection/us-department-transportation-service-animal) confirming the animal can relieve itself in a sanitary manner if the flight is eight or more hours. Airlines cannot require other documentation except to comply with transport regulations.

TRAVELING WITH A SERVICE ANIMAL
At the airport, request information on the nearest service animal relief areas. Onboard, service animals must fit under the seat in front of you or sit on your lap if small enough. They cannot block aisles or access to emergency exits and must behave properly.

Traveling outside the United States
When traveling internationally, verify if your destination country permits your service animal and what requirements are needed for legal entry and exit.

Encountering a Problem

If you believe your rights under the Air Carrier Access Act have been violated, request to speak with a Complaints Resolution Official (CRO). CROs are airline experts on disability accommodation issues and must be available at no cost, in person at the airport, or by telephone during operating hours.[2]

---

[2] "Service Animals," U.S. Department of Transportation (DOT), June 9, 2021. Available online. URL: www.transportation.gov/individuals/aviation-consumer-protection/service-animals. Accessed July 31, 2024.

Part 7 | Safety and Security Measures

Chapter 43 | Customs Restrictions and Regulations for Travelers

CUSTOMS RESTRICTIONS OF FOREIGN DESTINATIONS—WHAT YOU CANNOT TAKE TO OTHER COUNTRIES

Many countries restrict what you can bring into them. These restrictions may include items such as food, pets, and medications. Even some over-the-counter (OTC) medications are prohibited in certain countries. Check the country information page (https://travel.state.gov/content/travel/en/international-travel/International-Travel-Country-Information-Pages.html) at the U.S. Department of State's travel website for your destination to find contact information for its embassy or consulate in the United States.

CUSTOMS RESTRICTIONS IN FOREIGN DESTINATIONS—WHAT YOU CANNOT TAKE OUT OF OTHER COUNTRIES

Some countries may not allow you to take certain items out of the country. These items may include the following:
- currency
- gold and other precious metals
- precious and semi-precious stones
- electronic equipment not declared on arrival
- firearms and ammunition
- antiques
- animal skins
- religious artifacts and literature
- ivory and certain other wildlife parts and products

Countries may require export permits, which can take time to process. If you violate foreign customs rules, you may be detained at the airport and fined. You may also have your items confiscated and, in some cases, be prosecuted and/or sentenced to prison.

U.S. CUSTOMS RESTRICTIONS—WHAT YOU CANNOT BRING INTO THE UNITED STATES

There are certain items that you cannot bring into the United States, as well as items that are allowed only under specific conditions. Always check the latest information from official sources before your trip to ensure a smooth and hassle-free experience.[1]

Chapter 44 | Airport Security Screening

The Transportation Security Administration (TSA) incorporates unpredictable security measures, both seen and unseen, to accomplish its transportation security mission.

Security measures begin long before you arrive at the airport. TSA works closely with the intelligence and law enforcement communities to share information. Additional security measures are in place from when you get to the airport until you reach your destination.

The TSA adjusts processes and procedures to meet evolving threats and achieve the highest levels of transportation security. Because of this, you may notice changes in procedures from time to time.

The TSA counts on the traveling public to report unattended bags or packages, individuals possessing threatening items, persons trying to enter a restricted area, or similar suspicious activities at airports, train stations, bus stops, and ports. Report suspicious activity to local law enforcement.

Passenger screening at the airport is part of TSA's layered approach to security to get you safely to your destination. The TSA's screening procedures are intended to prevent prohibited items and other threats to transportation security from entering the sterile area of the airport and are developed in response to information on threats to transportation security.

CARRY-ON BAGGAGE SCREENING
Carry-On Baggage Screening in Standard Lanes
The TSA screens approximately 3.3 million carry-on bags for explosives and other dangerous items daily. Here is what to expect when taking your carry-on bag through security screening next time you fly.

Electronics

You will be asked to remove personal electronic devices larger than a cell phone from your carry-on bag and place them into a bin with nothing placed on or under them for x-ray screening. Common examples of these devices include laptops, tablets, e-readers, and handheld game consoles.

Note: *This does not include items such as hair dryers, electric shavers, or electric toothbrushes.*

Food

Listen to the instructions of the TSA officer. In most cases, food or snacks, such as fruit, health bars, and sandwiches can stay inside your carry-on bag. There are special instructions for liquids, gels, and aerosols, as well as for baby food, breast milk, and medically necessary items.

Note: *A TSA officer will be available to guide you through the process.*

Packing

If you are preparing for your flight, know how and what you pack can affect the screening process. Be sure to check for prohibited items and remember to follow the 3-1-1 liquids rule.

In addition to screening personal electronic devices separately, including laptops, tablets, e-readers, and handheld game consoles, TSA officers may instruct travelers to separate other items from carry-on bags, such as foods, powders, and any materials that can clutter bags and obstruct clear images on the x-ray machine. The TSA recommends keeping your bag organized to help ease the screening process, as it takes time for TSA officers to ensure a jam-packed, cluttered, and overstuffed bag is safe.

CHECKED BAGGAGE SCREENING

The TSA screens approximately 1.3 million checked bags for explosives and other dangerous items daily. Upon check-in, your checked baggage will be provided to the TSA for security screening. Once the screening process has been completed, your airline will transport your checked baggage to your respective flight and deliver it to the baggage-claim area. The majority of checked baggage is screened without the need for a physical bag search.

Inspection Notices
The TSA may inspect your checked baggage during the screening process. If your property is physically inspected, TSA will notice baggage inspection inside your bag. This is to inform you that an officer conducted an inspection of your property.

Claims
If your property is lost or damaged during the screening process, you may file a claim with TSA. If your property is lost or damaged during transport to the plane or baggage claim, please contact your airline.

Locks
The TSA has been provided universal "master" keys under agreements with Safe Skies Luggage Locks and Travel Sentry so that certain branded locks may not have to be cut to inspect baggage. These locks are commercially available, and the packaging on the locks should indicate that they may be opened by TSA officers. The TSA has no position on the validity or effectiveness of these products as a security measure and will be forced to remove them if necessary during the inspection.

Monitoring
Individual airports are responsible for access control and video monitoring of checked baggage facilities as part of their security plan. Monitoring methods vary from airport to airport and may include closed-circuit television (CCTV).

INTERNATIONAL FLIGHTS
The TSA works closely with international partners to maintain aviation security standards abroad.

The U.S. Department of Homeland Security (DHS) is actively working to raise the baseline for aviation security across the globe by requiring the implementation of enhanced security measures, both seen and unseen, at approximately 280 foreign airports with direct commercial flights to the United States in more than 100 countries around the world.

What to Expect

If you are flying from any of the last-point-of-departure airports into the United States, you may experience a more extensive screening process and should prepare for additional screening of your property and personal electronic devices. The TSA recommends arriving early at the airport to allow enough time for the screening process. Please know there are no changes to items allowed in carry-on and checked baggage.

For your convenience, the TSA encourages you to place powder-like substances over 12 oz./350 mL in your checked bags. Powders in carry-on baggage may require secondary screening, and powders that security officials cannot resolve will be prohibited from the cabin of the aircraft, effective June 30, 2018.

Note: *Check with your airline if you have questions about your flight to the United States.*

Electronics Restriction

There are currently no airlines under restrictions for large personal electronic devices.

Overseas Foods and Goods

Visit the U.S. Customs and Border Protection (CBP) Know Before You Go page (www.cbp.gov/travel/us-citizens/know-before-you-go) for information on what you can bring upon entry to the United States.

Hazardous Materials

Most hazardous materials are forbidden in carry-on and checked baggage. There are a few exceptions for some personal items, such as toiletries, medicines, battery-powered electronics, and assistive devices.

PAT-DOWN SCREENING

Pat-down procedures are used to determine whether prohibited items or other threats to transportation security are concealed on the person. You may be required to undergo a pat-down procedure if the screening technology alarms are triggered, as part of unpredictable security measures, for enhanced screening, or as an alternative to other types of screening, such as advanced imaging technology (AIT) screening. Even passengers who normally receive expedited screening, such as TSA PreCheck® passengers, may sometimes receive a pat-down.

A pat-down may include inspecting the head, neck, arms, torso, legs, and feet. This includes head coverings and sensitive areas, such as breasts, groin, and buttocks. You may be required to adjust clothing during the pat-down. The officer will advise you of the procedure to help you anticipate any actions before you feel them. Pat-downs require sufficient pressure to ensure detection, and areas may undergo a pat-down more than once for the TSA officer to confirm no threat items are detected.

The TSA officers use the back of their hands for pat-downs over sensitive areas of the body. In limited cases, additional screening involving a sensitive area pat-down with the front of the hand may be needed to determine that a threat does not exist.

You will receive a pat-down by an officer of the same gender. The TSA officers will explain the procedures to you as they conduct the pat-down. Please inform an officer if you have difficulty raising your arms, remaining in the position required, an external medical device, or areas of the body that are painful when touched. You may request a chair to sit if needed.

At any time during the process, you may request private screening accompanied by a companion of your choice. A second officer of the same gender will always be present during private screening.

SCREENING TECHNOLOGY

The TSA uses millimeter wave AIT and walk-through metal detectors to screen passengers. Millimeter wave AIT safely screens passengers without physical contact for metallic and nonmetallic threats, including weapons and explosives, which may be concealed under clothing. Generally, passengers undergoing screening can decline AIT screening in favor of physical screening. However, some passengers will be required to undergo AIT screening if their boarding pass indicates that they have been selected for enhanced screening, following TSA regulations, before their arrival at the security checkpoint. This will occur in a very limited number of circumstances. The vast majority of passengers will not be affected.

Safety

Advanced imaging technology is safe and meets national health and safety standards. This technology uses nonionizing radio-frequency energy in the millimeter spectrum with no known adverse health effects. It does not use x-ray technology.

Privacy

The TSA has strict privacy standards when using AIT to protect your privacy. Advanced imaging technology uses automated target recognition software that eliminates passenger-specific images and instead auto-detects potential threats by indicating their location on a generic outline of a person. The generic outline is identical for all passengers.

Light Outer Garment/Bulky Clothing

Any individual wearing a light outer garment or bulky clothing, when screened through AIT, will be asked to divest their light outerwear or bulky clothing. A light outer garment is defined as an outer layer of clothing that has a full front zipper or buttons used to fasten the outer garment, excluding button shirts. Examples include but are not limited to windbreakers and vests, suit/sport coats, blazers, and light jackets. Bulky clothing is a garment that is very loose or does not conform to the contour of the person. Examples include but are not limited to oversize pullover hoodies, large sweaters, cardigans, and ponchos. If an individual cannot or is not willing to remove a light outer garment or bulky clothing, let the officer know, and additional screening may occur.

SECURE FLIGHT

Secure Flight is a risk-based passenger prescreening program that enhances security by identifying low- and high-risk passengers before they arrive at the airport by matching their names against trusted traveler lists and watchlists.

To protect privacy, the Secure Flight program collects the minimum amount of personal information, such as full name, date of birth, and gender, necessary to conduct effective matching. Read the Privacy Impact Assessment (PIA; www.dhs.gov/publication/dhstsapia-018-tsa-secure-flight) and the System of Records Notice (SORN; www.govinfo.gov/content/pkg/FR-2015-01-05/html/2014-30856.htm) for information about the program's rigorous privacy protections. Personal data is collected, used, distributed, stored, and disposed of according to stringent guidelines.

Secure Flight transmits the screening instructions back to the airlines to identify low-risk passengers eligible for TSA PreCheck®; individuals on the Selectee List who are designated for enhanced screening; and those who will receive standard screening. Secure Flight also prevents individuals on the No Fly List and Centers for Disease Control and Prevention (CDC) Do Not Board List from boarding an aircraft. The Travel Redress Program (www.tsa.gov/travel/security-screening/travel-redress-program) resolves travel-related screening or inspection issues.

STANDARD AND TSA PRECHECK® SCREENING

The standard screening requires that you remove all items and place them on the x-ray belt for screening. With TSA PreCheck®, you can speed through security and do not need to remove your shoes, laptops, liquids, belts, and light jackets. Learn how to receive expedited screening with TSA PreCheck® (www.tsa.gov/precheck).

Note: *The TSA uses unpredictable security measures throughout the airport, and no individual is guaranteed expedited screening.*[1]

---

[1] "Security Screening," Transportation Security Administration (TSA), June 30, 2018. Available online. URL: www.tsa.gov/travel/security-screening. Accessed August 1, 2024.

Chapter 45 | Cybersecurity Tips for International Travelers

When traveling internationally, remember that your mobile phone and other personal communication devices transmit and store your personal information, which is as valuable as the contents of your suitcase, if not more so.

BEFORE YOU GO

Take proactive steps to secure your devices and your personally identifiable information (such as your name, address, date of birth, and Social Security Number (SSN)) before you travel. Leave at home any electronic equipment you do not need during your trip. If you take it, protect it. Be sure to:

- back up your electronic files
- remove sensitive data
- install strong passwords
- confirm antivirus software is up-to-date

WHILE TRAVELING

Be vigilant about your surroundings and where and how you use your devices. Make sure to:

- keep your devices secure in public places such as airports, hotels, and restaurants
- take care that nobody is trying to steal information from you by spying on your device screen while it is in use

- consider using a privacy screen on your laptop to restrict visibility

BE CAUTIOUS WHILE USING PUBLIC WI-FI

Some threats—such as device theft—are obvious. Others, though, may be invisible, such as data thieves attempting to steal passwords to compromise your personally identifiable information or access your accounts. You may be especially vulnerable in locations with public Wi-Fi, including Internet cafes, coffee shops, bookstores, travel agencies, clinics, libraries, airports, and hotels. Some helpful tips:

- Do not use the same passwords or personal identification numbers (PINs) abroad that you use in the United States.
- Avoid using public Wi-Fi to make online purchases or access bank accounts.
- Shut off your phone's auto-join function when logging into any public network.
- Periodically disconnect from and reconnect to public Wi-Fi networks while using them.
- Try purposely logging onto the public Wi-Fi with the wrong password. If you can still get on, that is a sign that the network is not secure.

Remember also to avoid using public equipment—such as phones, computers, and fax machines—for sensitive communications.

WHEN YOU GET HOME

Electronics and devices used or obtained abroad can be compromised. Your mobile phone and other electronic devices may be vulnerable to malware if you connect with local networks abroad. Update your security software and change your passwords on all devices when you return home.[1]

---

[1] "Cybersecurity Tips for International Travelers," Federal Communications Commission (FCC), January 15, 2021. Available online. URL: www.fcc.gov/consumers/guides/cybersecurity-tips-international-travelers. Accessed August 1, 2024.

Chapter 46 | **Recognizing and Preventing Scams While Traveling**

You can become the victim of a scam at home or abroad. There are many different types of scams, but they all share a common goal: taking your money. If someone is claiming to be your friend or relative in trouble overseas, the U.S. Embassy or Consulate may be able to help.

Before sending money, please review the tips.

TIPS TO PROTECT YOURSELF—AND YOUR MONEY— FROM SCAMS

- Before traveling abroad, research your destination.
- Generally, never send money to someone overseas if you have not met them in person—especially if you met online.
- Do not disclose personal details over the phone or online—even in your social media.
- Be aware that something that seems too good to be true usually is.
- Tell the person claiming to be a U.S. citizen in distress overseas to contact the nearest U.S. Embassy or Consulate.
- If someone claims to be a U.S. citizen overseas and says the embassy will not help, call the U.S. Department of State's (DOS) Overseas Citizens Services (OCS) at 888-407-4747. They can help you verify if the situation is real or a scam.
- If you send money to a U.S. citizen in an emergency through the DOS "OCS Trust" program, the person will need to show a photo ID to get the cash.

- If you have been the victim of a scam, file a complaint with the Federal Trade Commission (FTC) and the Federal Bureau of Investigation (FBI) at ic3.gov.

EXAMPLES OF COMMON SCAMS
Romance Scam
A person you have not met in person quickly offers friendship, romance, and/or marriage. They then claim to have problems overseas and ask for money. These scammers may say they need help paying hospital bills, visa fees, or legal expenses, among other examples.

Grandparent/Relative Scam
A person contacts you by email or social media, pretending to be your grandchild, niece, nephew, or other family member. They claim to need money right away, and usually ask you to keep it a secret. If this happens to you, find another way to contact the family member directly and confirm the facts.

Drug Trafficking Scam
These scams may begin as romantic relationships, or a scammer may contact you by phone or email to ask for help transporting something. They may offer a job abroad or the chance to do charity work. They may offer to pay for your travel or give you free luggage. They may also ask you to stop in another country to pick something up. They are very likely trying to get you to transport something illegal—such as drugs—in the hope you will not be detected, or so that when you are, it will be you and not them who face arrest. If someone asks you to transport something to another country, or back to the United States, be careful. Report it to airline and border authorities before you travel.

Lottery Scam
This scammer claims you have won a foreign lottery. They promise you a lot of prize money but tell you that you must first pay taxes and other processing fees. If you did not purchase a lottery ticket in a foreign country, you probably did not win a prize.

Wallet/Money Drop Scam

You see a wallet or cash on the ground. A scammer picks it up and shows you that it contains money. The scammer asks if the wallet belongs to you and tries to get you to touch it. Another scammer comes up and says the wallet is theirs. They accuse you of trying to steal it. The two scammers then threaten to call the police unless you pay them. In another version, the scammers ask to see your money to prove they did not steal it. When you take out your money, the scammers grab it and run away.

Teahouse/Restaurant/Bar Scam

An attractive young "English student" offers to show you around town. Then, they invite you to share a meal. You may be taken to a dimly lit back room or given a menu with small print. Your drinks may be spiked with drugs to impair your vision and judgment. When the bill comes, your host leaves, and you are left with a very expensive bill. The restaurant may threaten assault if you do not pay.

Arthouse/Rug Sale Scam

Someone claiming to be an art student will approach visitors at tourist sites. They will ask if you would like to see artwork created by local students and invite you to an art studio or gallery. They will share food and drink while introducing their art. Then, they will pressure you to buy artwork as compensation for their hospitality. Rug shops may use the same tactics.

Airport/"Bag Watching" Scam

A stranger asks you to watch their bag or purse. They leave and then return with someone posing as a police officer. The bag they left you with may contain drugs or other illegal items. The perpetrators then demand you give them money to avoid arrest.

Shell/Card Games

Scammers set up a game in popular tourist spots. They use three shells (or cups) with a small ball under one. They move the shells and then ask the audience to bet on which one the ball is under. People in the audience working with the scammers guess correctly the first few times. Then they let tourists join in. The tourists are allowed to win and bet more and more money. But then the scammer secretly takes the ball and the tourists lose—sometimes hundreds of dollars.[1]

[1] Bureau of Consular Affairs, "Protecting Yourself from Scams," U.S. Department of State (DOS), February 12, 2024. Available online. URL: https://travel.state.gov/content/travel/en/international-travel/emergencies/international-financial-scams.html. Accessed August 1, 2024.

Chapter 47 | **Replacing a Lost or Stolen Passport Abroad**

WHAT SHOULD YOU DO IF YOU LOSE YOUR PASSPORT WHILE TRAVELING?

You will have to replace the passport before returning to the United States. Contact the nearest U.S. Embassy or Consulate for assistance. Contact information for embassies and consulates is also available on this web page (https://travel.state.gov/content/travel/en/international-travel/International-Travel-Country-Information-Pages.html). Ask to speak to the Consular Section to report your passport lost or stolen.

You must appear in person at the U.S. Embassy or Consulate to apply for a new passport. If you are scheduled to leave the foreign country soon, please provide consular staff with the details of your travel. If there is not enough time to get you a regular passport, the Consular Section may be able to issue a limited-validity emergency passport, which may be valid for up to one year.

If a loved one informs you that their U.S. passport was lost or stolen overseas, you can call the Office of Overseas Citizens Services at 888-407-4747. They will help you connect your loved one with the closest U.S. Embassy or Consulate.

WHAT DO YOU NEED TO REPLACE YOUR PASSPORT OVERSEAS?

Please bring the following items to the embassy/consulate:
- one passport photo (obtaining it in advance can expedite the replacement process)

- identification (such as a driver's license or expired passport)
- evidence of U.S. citizenship (like a birth certificate or a photocopy of your missing passport)
- travel itinerary (airline/train tickets)
- DS-11 application for passport (https://travel.state.gov/content/travel/en/passports/how-apply/forms.html)
- DS-64 statement regarding a lost or stolen passport

Even if you cannot provide all of these documents, consular staff will assist you in quickly getting a new passport.

Police Report
A police report is not mandatory but can help confirm the circumstances of the loss or theft. If you lose your U.S. passport, we recommend notifying the local police. However, you may skip the report if you are concerned about delaying your travel.

HOW LONG IS A REPLACEMENT PASSPORT VALID?
Passports are valid for 10 years for adults and five years for minors. Need a quick fix for urgent travel? Get a limited-validity emergency passport, which is valid for up to one year. You can exchange it for a full-validity passport after your trip. You may also receive a limited passport if you have lost multiple passports or borrowed money from the State Department to fund your trip home. A consular officer can provide additional information.

ARE FEES CHARGED TO REPLACE LOST/STOLEN PASSPORTS ABROAD?
Replacement passports cost the same as any other passport. If you cannot pay for a new passport, you can provide consular staff with the names of people who might assist you.

If you have been a victim of a serious crime or disaster and cannot afford a new passport, you may be eligible for a free limited-validity emergency passport. If you want a full-validity passport, the regular fee applies for replacements.

CAN THE U.S. EMBASSY ISSUE A REPLACEMENT PASSPORT ON A WEEKEND OR HOLIDAY?

Most U.S. Embassies and Consulates cannot issue passports on weekends or holidays. However, they all have after-hours duty officers available to assist with life-or-death emergencies involving U.S. citizens abroad. Contact the nearest U.S. Embassy or Consulate's after-hours duty officer for help in emergencies, such as if you need to travel urgently or have been the victim of a serious crime. In most cases, a replacement passport will be issued the next business day.

CAN YOU TRAVEL IF YOU FIND YOUR PASSPORT AFTER REPORTING IT LOST OR STOLEN?

No. Once you report your passport lost or stolen, it is no longer valid for international travel. A foreign country may deny your entry if you attempt to use that passport, or you may be prevented from leaving if you are already abroad. If you wish to travel after reporting your passport lost or stolen, you must apply for a new passport.

By being prepared and informed, you can handle the loss of a passport efficiently and continue your travels with minimal disruption.[1]

---

[1] Bureau of Consular Affairs, "Lost or Stolen Passports Abroad," U.S. Department of State (DOS), March 8, 2024. Available online. URL: https://travel.state.gov/content/travel/en/international-travel/emergencies/lost-stolen-passport-abroad.html. Accessed August 1, 2024.

Chapter 48 | **Health Precautions for Animal-Related Risks and Insect Bites**

AVOID ANIMALS

Animals can look cute and cuddly, and you may want to pet them. However, any animal, whether friendly or harmless, can spread disease and may be dangerous.

While traveling, it is best to stay away from all animals. Any animal can bite, scratch, kick, or otherwise injure you, even if you did nothing to provoke it. Animals are often frightened of humans, trying to protect their territory or their young. Some diseases cause animals to behave aggressively toward people, even if they were previously friendly.

Check Your Destination for Animal-Related Health Risks

Before your trip, talk to your doctor about your planned activities. Find out what vaccines, medicines, or advice you may need to help prevent animal-related diseases at your destination.

Animals and Disease

When traveling, do not pet or feed animals, even pets, as they may not be vaccinated against rabies and other diseases. Animal licks and bites can cause bacterial infections that may require antibiotics, so seek medical attention after any contact with an animal. Also, ensure you are up-to-date on your tetanus vaccination.

- **Monkeys can spread rabies, Ebola, Marburg, herpes B virus, and tuberculosis**. If you are traveling to places where monkeys roam, do not touch or feed the monkeys.
- **Rodents, such as rats and mice, can spread many diseases through bites and scratches, urine, feces, or fleas that live on them**. These diseases include plague, leptospirosis, hantavirus disease, and rickettsial diseases. Avoid places with evidence of rodent activity, such as droppings or nesting materials. Do not touch anything that may be contaminated with rodent urine or feces.
- **Bats can spread rabies, as well as histoplasmosis, Ebola disease, and Marburg virus disease**. Stay away from caves, tunnels, or mines where bats live.
- **Birds can spread avian influenza and psittacosis, also known as "parrot fever."** Wash your hands with running water and soap after contact with birds or their droppings. If possible, avoid visiting poultry farms, bird markets, or other places where live poultry are raised, kept, or sold.

Rabies

Rabies is a deadly disease caused by a virus. It can be contracted by being bitten or scratched by an animal with rabies. If not promptly treated, rabies is almost always fatal. In many other parts of the world, rabies is a problem, and access to treatment is limited. These areas include much of Africa, Asia, Central America, and South America.

Traveling with Children

Watch young children carefully around unfamiliar animals. Children are more likely to be bitten, scratched, and seriously injured. Before travel, your child's health-care provider may recommend the rabies vaccine.

Act Quickly If an Animal Bites or Scratches You

- **Immediately wash all bites and scratches well.** Use plenty of soap and running water.
- **Seek medical care immediately.** Even if you do not feel sick or the wound does not look serious, infections and other complications can occur quickly.
- **To prevent rabies, start prophylaxis (preventive treatment) immediately after you have been bitten or scratched.** This includes getting a series of vaccines. Even if you were vaccinated against rabies before your trip, you still need to seek care and receive additional vaccine doses if you get bitten or scratched by an animal.
- **Be prepared to travel back to the United States or to another area to receive treatment.** Vaccination and medicine for rabies exposure are not available everywhere in the world.

After Travel

If you traveled and feel sick, particularly if you have a fever, talk to a health-care provider and inform them about any areas you recently traveled to.[1]

AVOID BUG BITES

Bugs, including mosquitoes, ticks, and fleas, can spread diseases such as malaria, yellow fever, Zika, dengue, chikungunya, and Lyme. While some cases are mild, these diseases can be severe and have lasting consequences. Some diseases caused by bug bites can be prevented with vaccines or medication, such as yellow fever and malaria; however, many cannot, such as Zika and Lyme. Learn more about steps you can take to avoid bug bites.

Check Your Destination

Your destination and activities may determine what steps you need to take to protect yourself from bug bites. Check the Centers for

---

[1] "Avoid Animals," Centers for Disease Control and Prevention (CDC), May 20, 2024. Available online. URL: wwwnc. cdc.gov/travel/page/be-safe-around-animals. Accessed August 1, 2024.

Disease Control and Prevention's (CDC) Destination (wwwnc.cdc. gov/travel/destinations/list) to see what vaccines or medicines you may need and what diseases or health risks are a concern at your destination.

Your Activities Can Increase Your Risk for Bug Bites

Some activities put you more at risk for bug bites than others. Activities that can increase your chances of getting bug bites include hiking, camping, working with animals, and visiting farms and forested areas.

Prevent Tick Bites

- **Know where to expect ticks**. Ticks live in grassy, brushy, or wooded areas or on animals. Spending time outside camping, gardening, or hunting could bring you in close contact with ticks. Many people get ticks in their own yards or neighborhoods.
- **Treat clothing and gear with products containing 0.5 percent permethrin**. Permethrin can be used to treat boots, clothing, and camping gear and remains protective through several washings. Alternatively, you can buy permethrin-treated clothing and gear.
- **Use U.S. Environmental Protection Agency (EPA)-registered insect repellents**. Use insect repellents such as N,N-diethyl-meta-toluamide (DEET), picaridin, IR3535, oil of lemon eucalyptus (OLE), para-menthane-diol (PMD), or 2-undecanone. EPA's search tool (www.epa.gov/insect-repellents/find-repellent-right-you) can help you find the product that best suits your needs. Always follow product instructions. Do not use products containing OLE or PMD on children under three years old.
- Avoid contact with ticks:
  - Avoid wooded and brushy areas with high grass and leaf litter.
  - Walk in the center of trails.

Find and Remove Ticks

- **Check your clothing for ticks**. Ticks may be carried into the house on clothing. Any ticks that are found should be removed. When possible, tumble dry clothes in a dryer on high heat for 10 minutes to kill ticks on dry clothing after you come indoors. If the clothes are damp, additional time may be needed. If the clothes require washing first, hot water is recommended. Cold and medium-temperature water will not kill ticks.
- **Examine gear and pets**. Ticks can ride on clothing and pets, then attach to a person later, so carefully examine pets, coats, and daypacks.
- **Shower soon after being outdoors**. Showering within two hours of coming indoors has been shown to reduce your risk of getting tick-borne diseases. Showering may help wash off unattached ticks and is a good opportunity to do a tick check.
- **Check your body for ticks**. Conduct a full-body check upon return from potentially tick-infested areas. Use a hand-held or full-length mirror to view all parts of your body. Check these parts of your body for ticks:
  - under the arms
  - in and around the ears
  - inside the belly button
  - back of the knees
  - in and around the hair
  - between the legs
  - around the waist

If you find a tick attached to your skin, remove it as soon as possible.

Keep Mosquitoes Out of Your Hotel Room or Lodging

- Choose a hotel or lodging with air conditioning or window and door screens.
- Use a mosquito net if you cannot stay in a place with air conditioning or window and door screens or if you are sleeping outside.

Sleep under a Mosquito Net

- If you are outside or when screened rooms are not available, sleep under a mosquito net. Mosquitoes can live indoors and bite during the day and night.
- Buy a mosquito net at your local outdoor store or online before traveling overseas.
- Choose a mosquito net that is compact, white, rectangular, with 156 holes per square inch, and long enough to tuck under the mattress.
- Permethrin-treated mosquito nets provide more protection than untreated nets.

After Travel

If you traveled and feel sick, particularly if you have a fever, talk to a health-care provider and inform them about any areas you recently traveled to.[2]

[2] "Avoid Bug Bites," Centers for Disease Control and Prevention (CDC), May 11, 2022. Available online. URL: wwwnc.cdc.gov/travel/page/avoid-bug-bites. Accessed August 1, 2024.

Chapter 49 | **Eating and Drinking Safely While Traveling**

Contaminated food or drinks may cause travelers' diarrhea and other diseases, disrupting your travel. Learn how to incorporate safer eating and drinking habits to reduce your chances of getting sick when you travel. Always wash your hands with soap and water before eating and preparing food. If soap and water are not readily available, use an alcohol-based hand sanitizer that contains at least 60 percent alcohol.

FOOD CONSIDERATIONS WHEN TRAVELING

- **Avoid lukewarm food**. Cold food should be served cold, and hot food should be served hot. If you select food from a buffet or salad bar, ensure the hot food is steaming, and the cold food is chilled. Germs that cause food poisoning grow quickly when food is in the danger zone, between 40 °F (4.44 °C) and 140 °F (60 °C).
- **Dry or packaged foods**. Most germs require a damp environment to grow, so dry foods, such as potato chips, are usually safe. Additionally, food in factory-sealed containers, such as canned tuna or packaged crackers, is generally safe if it has not been opened or handled by another person.
- **Baby formula**. If preparing baby formula, use a safe water source per the guidance below. See safety guidance for formula preparation and storage.

- **Avoid raw foods**. Fruits or vegetables may be safer to eat if you can peel them yourself or wash them in bottled or disinfected water.
  - Stay away from cut-up fruit or vegetables. They may have been contaminated during preparation.
  - Avoid eating fresh salads, even if finely cut or shredded. They may be contaminated with human or animal waste that even clean water cannot wash off.
  - Avoid fresh salsas, condiments, and other sauces made from raw fruits or vegetables.
  - Avoid eating raw meat or seafood, including items "cooked" with citrus juice, vinegar, or other acidic liquids (such as ceviche).
- **Street food**. Avoid eating food from street vendors. If you choose to eat street food, follow the same food safety rules as you would with other foods. For example, avoid raw vegetables and eat food cooked and steaming hot.
- **Avoid bushmeat**. Bushmeat refers to local wild game, generally animals not typically eaten in the United States, such as bats, monkeys, or rodents. Bushmeat can be a source of animal-to-human transmission of diseases, such as Ebola.

DRINK CONSIDERATIONS WHEN TRAVELING

- **Tap water**. Do not drink the tap water in countries where it might be contaminated. Avoid swallowing water when showering, and brush your teeth with bottled or disinfected water. Tap water can be disinfected by boiling, filtering, or chemically treating it.
  - When visiting places with unknown water quality, treat your water to ensure it is safe to drink.
- **Ice**. Do not use ice in destinations with limited access to clean water or where there is concern about contaminated drinking water, as it was likely made with tap water.
- **Bottled or canned drinks**. Drinks from unopened, factory-sealed bottles or cans are safer than tap water; however, use caution as vendors in some countries may

replace bottled water with untreated water. Sometimes, a drop of glue can mimic the factory seal. Carbonated drinks in bottles or cans, such as sodas or sparkling water, are typically safe because the bubbles indicate that the bottle was sealed at the factory and not tampered with. Avoid drinks with ice.

- **Hot drinks**. Hot coffee or tea should be safe if served steaming hot. It is okay to let it cool before drinking. Do not drink coffee or tea served warm or at room temperature. Be careful about adding potentially contaminated items to your hot drinks, such as cream or lemon. Sugar is usually safe because it is a dry food.
- **Milk**. Pasteurized milk from a sealed bottle is usually safe to drink. Do not drink milk stored in open containers, such as pitchers, that may have been sitting at room temperature; this includes cream for coffee or tea. Unpasteurized foods carry risks for all travelers; however, it is especially important for pregnant women or people with weakened immune systems to avoid unpasteurized milk, cheese, and yogurt.
- **Alcohol**. The alcohol content of most liquors kills germs that may have been present. When choosing mixers, such as fruit juices, follow the recommendations about what types of food and drink are least likely to harbor germs. Avoid drinks with ice.
- **Fountain drinks**. Sodas from a fountain, such as those in restaurants, are made by carbonating water and mixing it with flavored syrup. Since the water most likely came from the restaurant's tap, do not drink fountain drinks.
- **Freshly squeezed juice**. Avoid fruit juice, and food and drinks made with freshly squeezed juice made by others. It is fine to drink fruit juice or eat ice pops and other treats if you washed/peeled the fruit in bottled or treated water and squeezed the juice yourself.[1]

---

[1] "Food and Drink Considerations When Traveling," Centers for Disease Control and Prevention (CDC), July 13, 2023. Available online. URL: wwwnc.cdc.gov/travel/page/food-water-safety. Accessed August 1, 2024.

Chapter 50 | **Protecting Yourself from Counterfeit Drugs Abroad**

AVOIDING COUNTERFEIT DRUGS

The best way to avoid counterfeit drugs is to reduce the need to purchase medications abroad. Travelers should be instructed to purchase anticipated amounts of medications for chronic conditions (e.g., arthritis, diabetes, hypertension), medications for travelers' diarrhea, and prophylactic medications for infectious diseases (e.g., malaria) before traveling. It is advisable to avoid buying drugs online, as the source of the medication often cannot be verified. Travelers should also be aware that other health-related items obtained abroad (e.g., medical devices, insect repellents, mosquito nets) could also be counterfeit, falsified, or substandard.

PREPARING FOR INTERNATIONAL TRAVEL

In preparation for international travel, travelers should obtain all necessary medicines and other health-related items before the trip. Prescriptions written in the United States usually cannot be filled overseas, and although many U.S. prescription medications are available for over-the-counter (OTC) purchases in foreign countries, some might not be available at all. Since checked baggage can get lost, travelers should pack medications and first aid items in a carry-on bag and bring extra medicine in case of travel delays. Medications should be carried in their original containers, with the patient's name and dosage regimen appearing on the container for prescription drugs. Travelers should also bring the "patient prescription information" sheet, which provides information on common generic and brand names, use, side effects, precautions, and drug interactions. It is crucial to check with the embassies of destination countries for prohibited drugs, as many countries have restrictions on medicines, including OTC medications, entering their borders.

ENSURING MEDICATION SAFETY

If travelers run out of and require additional medications, they should take steps to ensure the medicines they buy are safe (see Table 50.1 for a list of online resources). One way to ensure medication safety is by comparing distinguishing features of the packaging, especially when authentic packaging is unavailable or if the traveler is not familiar with the brand. For example, the batch and lot numbers, manufacturing date, and expiration date printed on the outside of the box should match those on the insert or blister pack.

Table 50.1. Online Resources for Travelers Purchasing Medicines and Medical Products Overseas

Organization/Source	Resource
Drugs.com	Pill Identifier (www.drugs.com/pill_identification.html)
International Society of Travel Medicine (ISTM)	Database on International Regulations on Importation of Medicines for Personal Use (www.istmfoundation.net/Files/Images/Activities/ISTM%20database%20on%20International%20regulations%20explanation%208%20Aug%202018.pdf)
Transportation Security Administration (TSA)	Disabilities and Medical Conditions (www.tsa.gov/travel/tsa-cares)
Centers for Disease Control and Prevention (CDC)	Counterfeit Medicines (wwwnc.cdc.gov/travel/page/counterfeit-medicine)
U.S. Customs and Border Protection (CBP)	Prohibited and Restricted Items (see Medication; www.cbp.gov/travel/us-citizens/know-before-you-go/prohibited-and-restricted-items)
U.S. Food and Drug Administration (FDA)	Drug Safety and Availability (www.fda.gov/drugs/drug-safety-and-availability)
U.S. Pharmacopeia (USP)	Medicines Quality Database (MQDB; www.usp.org/global-public-health/medicines-quality-database)
World Health Organization (WHO)	Substandard and Falsified Medical Products (www.who.int/news-room/fact-sheets/detail/substandard-and-falsified-medical-products)

PURCHASING MEDICINES OVERSEAS: A GOOD PRACTICES CHECKLIST FOR INTERNATIONAL TRAVELERS

- **Obtain medicines from a legitimate pharmacy**. The local U.S. Embassy or Consulate might help locate legitimate local pharmacies. Do not buy from open markets, street vendors, or suspicious-looking pharmacies; request a receipt when purchasing.
- **Do not buy medicines priced substantially lower than the typical price**. Although generic medications are usually less expensive, many counterfeit brand names are sold at prices significantly lower than normal.
- **Ensure the medicines are in their original packages or containers**. If you receive medicines as loose tablets or capsules in a plastic bag or envelope, ask the pharmacist to show you the container from which the medicine was dispensed. Record the brand, batch number, and expiration date. Sometimes a wary consumer will prompt the seller to supply quality medicine rather than a counterfeit or substandard one.
- **Be familiar with your medications**. The size, shape, color, and taste of counterfeit medicines might differ from the authentic product. Discoloration, splits, cracks, spots, and stickiness of tablets or capsules are indications of possible counterfeit. These defects may also indicate improper storage. Keep examples of authentic medications to compare if you purchase the same brand.
- **Be familiar with the packaging**. Different color inks, poor-quality printing or packaging materials, and misspelled words are clues to counterfeit drugs. Keep an example of packaging for comparison and observe the expiration date.

Always consult with health-care professionals and local authorities for the best practices in obtaining and using medications during international travel.[1]

---

[1] "Perspectives: Avoiding Poorly Regulated Medicines and Medical Products during Travel," Centers for Disease Control and Prevention (CDC), May 1, 2023. Available online. URL: wwwnc.cdc.gov/travel/yellowbook/2024/health-care-abroad/avoiding-poorly-regulated-medicines-and-medical-products. Accessed August 1, 2024.

Chapter 51 | **Drug and Alcohol Awareness for Travelers**

OBEY LOCAL LAWS AND REGULATIONS REGARDING DRUGS AND ALCOHOL

When traveling overseas, it is crucial to obey the laws and regulations of the country you are visiting, especially those pertaining to drug and alcohol use. Every year, many American students are arrested abroad on drug charges or because of their behavior under the influence.

AVOID UNDERAGE AND EXCESSIVE ALCOHOL CONSUMPTION

Many arrests, accidents, and violent crimes have occurred as a result of alcohol abuse. While abroad, driving under the influence and drinking on the street or on public transportation may be considered criminal activities by local authorities, as they would be in many places in the United States.

ENSURE YOUR PRESCRIPTION MEDICATION IS NOT CONSIDERED AN ILLEGAL NARCOTIC

If you are going abroad with a preexisting medical condition, carry a letter from your doctor describing your condition and medications, including the generic names of prescribed drugs. Any medications carried overseas should be in their original containers and clearly labeled. Check with the foreign country's embassy in the United States to ensure your medications are not considered illegal narcotics.

DO NOT ACCEPT PACKAGES FROM ANYONE

Some Americans think it is a good idea to take advantage of an offer for an all-expense-paid vacation abroad in exchange for carrying a small package in their luggage. However, ignorance is no excuse if you are caught. If the package contains illegal drugs or substances, the fact that you did not know will not reduce the charges. You could miss your flight, your exams, or several years of your life during a stay behind bars.

DO NOT IMPORT, PURCHASE, USE, OR POSSESS DRUGS

Drug charges can carry severe consequences, including imprisonment without bail for up to a year and sentences ranging from fines to jail time. Some crimes even carry the death penalty. Contraband or paraphernalia associated with illegal drug use can also get you in trouble.[1]

---

[1] Bureau of Consular Affairs, Alcohol and Drugs Overseas," U.S. Department of State (DOS), December 2007. Available online. URL: https://travel.state.gov/content/dam/students-abroad/pdfs/alcohol.pdf. Accessed August 1, 2024.

Chapter 52 | **Sexual Health and Safety While Traveling**

About one in three travelers will have sex with a new partner while on a trip. The excitement of being in another country and meeting new people may lead travelers to engage in risky behaviors that can lead to sexually transmitted infections (STIs), including human immunodeficiency virus (HIV), gonorrhea, chlamydia, and syphilis. Some people travel for "sex tourism," which is defined as travel planned specifically for the purpose of sex, generally to a country where sex work is legal.

Sexually transmitted infections may occur without any signs or symptoms, so you may not realize that you or a partner is infected. While most STIs are treatable, some can cause serious health problems if left untreated.

The following activities put you at risk for STIs:
- having anal, vaginal, or oral sex without a condom
- having multiple sex partners
- having anonymous sex partners
- having sex while under the influence of drugs or alcohol, which can lower inhibitions and result in greater sexual risk-taking

TAKE STEPS TO PROTECT YOURSELF

Not having sex or having sex with one uninfected partner are the most reliable ways to avoid getting and spreading STIs. However, if you have sex with new partners during your trip, take steps to protect yourself and your partners.
- Use a new condom, consistently and correctly, for every act of vaginal, anal, and oral sex throughout the entire

sex act (from start to finish). Bring condoms from the
United States, because those in other countries may not
be up to U.S. quality standards.
- Get vaccinated for hepatitis A and hepatitis B before
you travel; both viruses can be spread through sex.
- Talk to your doctor about a human papillomavirus
(HPV) vaccine.
- If you are concerned about HIV, discuss pre-exposure
prophylaxis (PrEP) with your health-care provider.
PrEP is usually available as a pill or a shot.

SYMPTOMS OF SEXUALLY TRANSMITTED INFECTIONS
The symptoms of STIs vary depending on the infection. Many STIs
do not cause any symptoms at all. When symptoms do occur, they
may include:
- pain when you urinate or have sex
- discharge from the vagina, penis, or anus
- unexplained rash, sores, or ulcers on your skin,
genitals, or throat
- jaundice (yellow color of the skin and eyes)

SEEK TREATMENT EARLY
Treating STIs early is crucial to prevent more serious and long-term
complications and to avoid spreading infections to your partners. If
you are sexually active, talk to your health-care provider about getting tested for STIs. If you have symptoms, take the following steps:
- Do not have sex.
- See your health-care provider.
- Be open and honest with your provider, and inform them
about recent sexual history and international travel.
- If your provider diagnoses you with an STI, notify your
recent sex partners. They may also be infected and may
need to get tested and treated.[1]

[1] "Sexually Transmitted Infections," Centers for Disease Control and Prevention (CDC), September 15, 2022.
Available online. URL: wwwnc.cdc.gov/travel/page/std. Accessed August 1, 2024.

Chapter 53 | Support for U.S. Citizens Arrested Overseas

One of the highest priorities of the U.S. Department of State (DOS) and U.S. Embassies and Consulates abroad is to provide assistance to U.S. citizens incarcerated overseas. The DOS is committed to ensuring fair and humane treatment for U.S. citizens imprisoned abroad. The DOS stands ready to assist incarcerated citizens and their families within the limits of their authority, in accordance with international, domestic, and foreign law.

TIPS TO AVOID ARREST OVERSEAS

- Understand that you are subject to the local laws and regulations while visiting or living in a foreign country—follow them.
- Learn which laws might differ from those in the United States. The DOS provides information for each country on the Country Information page (https://travel.state.gov/content/travel/en/international-travel/International-Travel-Country-Information-Pages.html).

IN CASE OF AN ARREST OVERSEAS

- Ask the prison authorities to notify the U.S. Embassy or Consulate.
- Contact the closest U.S. Embassy or Consulate to inform the DOS about the arrest.

CONSULAR ASSISTANCE TO U.S. PRISONERS

When a U.S. citizen is arrested overseas, they may feel confused and disoriented, as they are in unfamiliar surroundings and may not know the local language, customs, or legal system.

The Bureau of Consular Affairs can:

- provide a list of local attorneys who speak English
- contact family, friends, or employers of the detained U.S. citizen (with their written permission)
- visit the detained U.S. citizen regularly and provide reading materials and vitamin supplements, where appropriate
- ensure that prison officials are providing appropriate medical care
- provide a general overview of the local criminal justice process
- upon request, ensure that prison officials permit visits with a member of the clergy of the detainee's choice
- establish an Overseas Citizens Services (OCS) Trust, if necessary, so friends and family can transfer funds to imprisoned U.S. citizens

The Bureau of Consular Affairs cannot:

- get U.S. citizens out of jail
- state to a court that anyone is guilty or innocent
- provide legal advice or represent U.S. citizens in court
- serve as official interpreters or translators
- pay legal, medical, or other fees[1]

---

[1] Bureau of Consular Affairs, "Arrest or Detention of a U.S. Citizen Abroad," U.S. Department of State (DOS), February 27, 2023. Available online. URL: https://travel.state.gov/content/travel/en/international-travel/emergencies/arrest-detention.html. Accessed August 1, 2024.

Chapter 54 | Safety Essentials for Camping in National Parks

CAMPING SAFELY

The goal is to ensure your safety while visiting a national park. As a visitor, you are responsible for your own safety. Please remember the following:

- Plan for your park visit. (Careful planning will prevent many safety issues.)
- Research and learn about possible risks in the park environment and your camping trip before you go.
- Seek and listen to the information, advice, and warnings provided by park staff.
- Know your physical and mental limits.
- Take action by using good judgment and selecting the right equipment and supplies to prevent any injuries during your visit.

BEFORE THE TRIP
Know Your Limits

Parks offer a wide variety of activities with different settings and levels of difficulty. When planning your trip, match the interests and physical fitness of your group with the activities you choose. Some families may prefer bird watching and easy hikes around a lake, while others may seek adventure in whitewater rafting or mountain climbing. It is important not to push yourself or group members beyond their physical abilities, as this increases the risk of injuries. If you have questions about your fitness level, health conditions, or appropriate activities, consult a doctor. Once everything is planned, enjoy the adventure!

Plan Your Trip

After determining your group's limits and experience level, choose the park you want to visit, explore camping options, and select your campsite. Consider the setting, time of year, and difficulty level to plan the right equipment before heading out.

- **Setting**. Consider the environment—whether it is a beach, desert, or forest.
- **Time of year**. Consider the season and potential weather conditions, such as heat, humidity, or cold and snow.
- **Difficulty level**. Assess how accessible the campsite is. Determine whether you can drive to the site or if hiking is required, and ensure everyone in the group can manage the hike.
- **Duration**. The length of your trip will determine the amount of food, clothing, and other supplies needed.

In Case of Emergency

The old saying, "Hope for the best, plan for the worst," applies to camping. Take steps to help emergency responders locate you in case of an emergency.

- **Emergency contact**. Designate a friend or family member not going on the trip as an emergency contact and leave your travel itinerary with them.
- **Travel itinerary**. Include the following information:
  - names and contact information of group members
  - description of your vehicle or boat, including make, model, and license plate number
  - starting time and location
  - details of your route and planned activities
  - types of equipment and supplies you have with you
  - expected finish time and location

- park's emergency phone number to call if you do not return on schedule

Leave your trip plan with your family and friends traveling with you, so they know the park's emergency numbers. This way, they can make contact in an emergency situation.

Prepare—Gear Up!

Identify your equipment needs based on the setting, time of year, difficulty, and trip duration. Here is a list of essential items:

- **Navigational supplies**. Include a map, GPS unit, and compass.
- **Sun and insect protection**. Pack sunscreen, a hat, insect repellent, and sunglasses.
- **Insulation**. Always bring extra clothing in case of cold weather conditions, precipitation, or wind.
- **Shelter**. Have an emergency shelter, such as a space blanket, bivvy, or tarp, whether on the trail or at camp.
- **Illumination**. Carry a flashlight or headlamp for visibility in the dark.
- **First aid kit**. Include all necessary medical supplies, from bandages to specialized medication for group members.
- **Fire**. Bring a fire starter, such as waterproof matches or a lighter.
- **Extra food and water**. Always carry more than you think you need.
- **Repair kits and tools**. Include items such as knives, multi-tools, and duct tape.
- **Communication device**. A cell phone is helpful, but consider bringing a personal locator beacon or satellite phone for optimal safety, as cell service may not be available.

UPON ARRIVAL

Reassess Group Health

Before beginning activities, check in with your group to assess their health and fitness. Any planned activities should align with the group's capabilities. Do not push yourself or others if they are not physically able. If someone is unwell, prioritize their care and avoid strenuous activities.

Ask a Park Ranger

If available, consult with a park ranger or campsite host for current information about outdoor conditions, regulations, and possible alerts. Ask about:

- **Environmental hazards**. Inquire about rock falls, fire, wildlife, high water in streams, or other conditions.
- **Weather**. Check for any forecasts of rain, wind, snow, or extreme temperatures that could affect your activities. Use local newspapers, weather-related websites, or radio stations for updates.
- **Park regulations**. Confirm rules about open fires, food disposal, and other regulations. Some parks may have fire bans or require food storage containers to prevent wildlife access.

DURING YOUR STAY
Set Up a Safe Camp

Follow guidelines for distances between food and sleeping areas, food storage and disposal, and other factors to ensure a safe camping experience.

- **Awareness of yourself, family, and friends**. Monitor the energy levels and health of group members. Know when to turn back, go to a backup plan, or end the trip. Consult a physician or other health-care professional if you have questions about fitness levels, health conditions, or required medications.
- **Awareness of your environment**. Be mindful of varying outdoor conditions, such as heat, cold, wetness, and dryness. Check for park alerts or conditions like wildlife sightings, severe weather, dead trees, rock falls, and air quality.

- **Ensure equipment is working properly.** Before engaging in activities like hiking or kayaking, check and test your equipment. Do not forget your essential items.
- **Drink water.** Stay hydrated by knowing where water sources are in the park and whether they are potable. Plan to haul or treat water if necessary.
- **Wear sun protection.** Use sunscreen to prevent sunburn. For extra protection, wear hats, long-sleeve shirts, and sunglasses.
- **Wear insect repellent.** Use bug spray to protect against mosquitoes, ticks, and other insects.
- **Dress in layers.** Adjust clothing as needed to stay comfortable and dry.
- **Wear boots.** Boots provide sturdy footing and help prevent ankle injuries.
- **Remove tripping hazards.** Clear the area around your site, especially in the cooking area, to avoid accidents.
- **Monitor the weather.** Stay aware of changing weather conditions.

Respect Wildlife

- **Do not feed wildlife.** Feeding animals can lead to persistent behavior and attract them to campsites.
- **Avoid contact with wildlife.** Keep a safe distance and do not approach animals.
- **Keep safe viewing distances.** Follow park guidelines for safe wildlife viewing distances.
- **Avoid attracting wildlife to your campsite.**

Keep Your Pet Safe, Too

- **Always keep your pet restrained.** Prevent them from wandering off or encountering wildlife.
- **Check your pet for ticks.** Check regularly to avoid tick-borne diseases.

- **Do not leave your pet in a closed vehicle**. It can quickly become dangerously hot.
- **Be cautious in bear country**. Camping with dogs in bear country can be dangerous, as dogs can attract bears.

AFTER THE TRIP

As your trip concludes, follow these steps to ensure a safe return home:

- Check in with your emergency contacts.
- Sign out of the logbook if you signed in at the beginning of your activity.
- Notify your emergency contact that you have safely concluded your trip.

Leave No Trace

- **Clean up your campsite**. Do not leave behind garbage, food scraps, or personal items.
- **Extinguish your campfire**. Double-check to confirm the fire is fully extinguished.
- **Properly dispose of garbage**. Follow park rules for trash disposal. Some parks may require carrying out garbage.

Assess the Outcome of the Trip and Any "Lessons Learned"

After each trip, review what went well and what could be improved. This reflection will help create a more enjoyable experience for future trips.

Share Your Experience

Share your experience and lessons learned to help others have a safe and enjoyable trip.[1]

---

[1] National Park Service (NPS), "Staying Safe—Camping," U.S. Department of the Interior (DOI), May 24, 2018. Available online. URL: www.nps.gov/subjects/camping/staying-safe.htm. Accessed August 1, 2024.

Chapter 55 | **Protecting Yourself from Terrorist Attacks**

Terrorist attacks often happen without warning. U.S. citizens should stay alert and take steps to enhance their security while traveling. Before your trip, check the Travel Advisories website (https://travel.state.gov) and sign up for the Smart Traveler Enrollment Program (STEP; step.state.gov), which sends security messages about threats. While abroad, stay informed by watching the local news and know the contact information for the nearest U.S. Embassy or Consulate.

Terrorist groups, their associates, and those inspired by them may target United States and Western citizens worldwide. Extremists may use conventional weapons or nontraditional ones but increasingly favor simpler methods to better target crowds. These methods include using edged weapons, pistols, and vehicles.

Extremists are increasingly attacking "soft" targets, which include:
- high-profile public events, such as sporting contests, political rallies, demonstrations, holiday events, celebratory gatherings, and so on.
- hotels, clubs, and restaurants
- places of worship
- schools
- parks
- shopping malls and markets
- tourism infrastructure
- public transportation systems
- airports

The recommendations below can help you avoid becoming a target. Following them may help deter would-be terrorists and provide peace of mind.

AIRPORTS AND AIR TRAVEL

- Schedule direct flights if possible. Avoid stops in high-risk airports or areas.
- Do not spend too much time in the public area of an airport. Move quickly from the check-in counter to security screening to enter the secured area. When you land, leave the airport as soon as possible, as arrival areas are typically less secure than departure areas.
- Watch for abandoned packages or other suspicious items. Report them to airport authorities and leave the area quickly.
- Avoid drawing attention to yourself as much as possible.

PUBLIC VENUES

- Avoid spending time at "soft" targets whenever possible. Be alert for suspicious or unusual activity.
- Be aware that Western-branded venues or Western-like facilities may be terrorist targets.
- Do not meet strangers at unknown or remote locations.
- Report suspicious activities and people to the local police and the nearest U.S. Embassy or Consulate.
- Identify potential safe areas, such as police stations, hotels, and hospitals. Formulate a plan of action and know where to go if a terrorist attack or security incident occurs.
- Remember the "run, hide, fight" rule during a terrorist attack or similar incident. If possible, quickly leave. If not, hide. As a last resort, if necessary, yell and fight.

TAXI CABS AND PERSONAL VEHICLES

- Travel with others if possible.
- Carry a charged cell phone at all times. Inform friends, family, and colleagues of your departures and arrivals.

- Select your own taxicab at random. Do not use an unlicensed cab. Taxis, Uber, or Uber-like vehicles should have photo licenses clearly displayed inside the vehicle or on the phone app. Compare the image and identifying information with the driver. Record the license plate information in your phone as a precaution.
- Inspect rental or personal vehicles for suspicious items or marks before driving.
- Drive with car windows closed whenever possible. Keep your vehicle in good operating condition with at least a half gasoline tank.

HOTELS

- Review evacuation and shelter-in-place plans for your hotel room.
- Know the identity of visitors before opening the door of your hotel room. Do not meet strangers in your hotel room.
- Refuse unexpected packages.
- Report suspicious activities to the hotel's front desk or security office.

POLICE AND SECURITY SERVICES

- Follow instructions provided by the police and security services during an emergency.[1]

---

[1] Bureau of Consular Affairs, "Terrorism," U.S. Department of State (DOS), March 6, 2024. Available online. URL: https://travel.state.gov/content/travel/en/international-travel/emergencies/terrorism.html. Accessed August 1, 2024.

Chapter 56 | **Dealing with Death Abroad**

The death of a friend, relative, or coworker can be immensely distressing, and the situation can be even more challenging when it occurs abroad. In such cases, grieving individuals may be unfamiliar with local laws, language, culture, and processes for investigation and the release of the body. Whether dealing with the death locally or from their home country, the next of kin may face large, unanticipated costs and labor-intensive administrative requirements.

Depending on the circumstances of the death, some countries require an autopsy. For travel companions of the deceased, as well as friends and relatives, sources of support might include the U.S. Consulate or Embassy, a travel insurance provider (particularly if coverage included repatriation of remains), the airline, a tour operator, faith-based and aid organizations, or the deceased person's employer. Official identification of the body will likely be necessary, and consular offices may need to issue official documents. A body can be identified through witness statements from those who knew the person well, DNA analysis, fingerprint checks, dental radiographs, or inspection of surgical implants.

DEATH ONBOARD A CONVEYANCE
Commercial Aircraft
Federal regulations require that all deaths aboard commercial flights and ships destined for the United States be reported to the Centers for Disease Control and Prevention (CDC). The Federal Aviation Administration (FAA) mandates that flight attendants receive training in cardiopulmonary resuscitation (CPR) and the

proper use of an automated external defibrillator (AED) at least once every two years. U.S. Good Samaritan laws protect actions taken in a medical emergency during flight unless there is gross negligence or willful misconduct.

If CPR is performed in an aircraft cabin for more than 30 minutes without signs of life and no shocks advised by an AED, the person may be presumed dead, and resuscitation efforts halted. Airlines may specify additional criteria for presuming death, depending on the availability of ground-to-air medical consultation services or a physician onboard. In these cases, the body should be secured and covered for the remainder of the flight.

Cruise Ships

If a death occurs on a cruise ship, the crew typically provides logistical support for repatriating the body. Cruise ships are equipped with morgues and body bags and are staffed with health-care professionals capable of providing clinical care. Any death involving an accident, violence, or foul play requires more extended and complicated processes. U.S. consular officials can provide general guidance and legal aid resource options. Some travel insurance products cover legal services abroad, so travelers should be aware of the exclusions and limitations of their policies.

OBTAINING U.S. DEPARTMENT OF STATE ASSISTANCE

When a U.S. citizen dies outside the United States, the deceased person's next of kin or legal representative should notify U.S. consular officials at the Department of State (DOS). Consular personnel are available 24/7 to assist U.S. citizens during overseas emergencies.

If the next of kin or legal representative is in a foreign country with the deceased U.S. citizen, they should contact the nearest U.S. Embassy or Consulate for assistance. Contact information for U.S. Embassies and Consulates overseas can be found on the DOS website (www.usembassy.gov).

Family members, domestic partners, or legal representatives in a different country from the deceased should call the DOS Office of Overseas Citizens Services in Washington, DC, at 888-407-4747 (toll-free) or 202-501-4444, Monday through Friday, 8 a.m. to 5 p.m.

Eastern time. For emergency assistance after hours or on weekends and holidays, call the DOS switchboard at 202-647-4000 and ask to speak with the Overseas Citizens Services duty officer. The nearest U.S. Embassy or Consulate to the country where the U.S. citizen died can also provide support.

The DOS does not provide funds for returning the remains of U.S. citizens who die abroad. U.S. consular officers assist the next of kin by conveying instructions to the appropriate offices within the foreign country and providing information on how to send the necessary private funds for preparing and repatriating the deceased person's remains. Upon issuance of a local (foreign) death certificate, the nearest U.S. Embassy or Consulate can prepare a consular report of the death of an American abroad. Copies of this report are provided to the next of kin or legal representative and can be used in U.S. courts to settle estate matters. If the deceased has no next of kin or legal representative in-country, a consular officer may act as a provisional conservator of the deceased person's personal effects.

IMPORTING HUMAN REMAINS FOR BURIAL, ENTOMBMENT, OR CREMATION

The CDC regulates the importation of human remains and provides guidance for their importation. The requirements are more stringent if the person dies from a disease classified as quarantinable in the United States.

Except for cremated remains, human remains intended for burial, entombment, or cremation after entry into the United States must be accompanied by a death certificate stating the cause of death. A death certificate is an official government document certifying a death has occurred and providing identifying information about the deceased, including (at a minimum) name, age, and sex. The document must also certify the time, place, and cause of death, if known. If the official government document is not written in English, it must be accompanied by an English translation attested by a person licensed to perform acts in legal affairs in the country where the death occurred.

In lieu of a death certificate, a copy of the Consular Mortuary Certificate and the Affidavit of Foreign Funeral Director and

Transit Permit together constitute acceptable identification of human remains. If a death certificate is not available in time for returning the remains, the U.S. Embassy or Consulate should provide a Consular Mortuary Certificate stating whether the person died from a disease classified as quarantinable in the United States. A person transporting human remains must also meet the requirements of the country of origin, air carrier, the Transportation Security Administration (TSA), and U.S. Customs and Border Protection (CBP).[1]

DEATH ABROAD
When a U.S. citizen dies abroad, the DOS is there to help.

First Steps
Hospitals or local police may notify the embassy or consulate of the death of a U.S. citizen. The DOS then attempts to locate and inform the next of kin of the U.S. citizen's death. The DOS can assist the next of kin by providing information, including details about local burial and other arrangements.

Disposition of Remains
The burial or cremation of a body must follow U.S. and foreign law. Options depend on the foreign country's facilities and local customs, which may differ significantly from those in the United States. The DOS has no funds to assist in returning the remains or ashes of U.S. citizens, but they can help convey instructions to the relevant offices in the foreign country and assist in sending private funds to cover overseas costs.

Consular Report of Death Abroad
After issuing a local (foreign) death certificate, the nearest embassy or consulate may prepare a Consular Report of Death Abroad (CRODA).

---

[1] "Death during Travel," Centers for Disease Control and Prevention (CDC), May 1, 2023. Available online. URL: wwwnc.cdc.gov/travel/yellowbook/2024/environmental-hazards-risks/death-during-travel. Accessed August 1, 2024.

Copies of this report are provided to the next of kin or legal representative and can be used in the United States to settle estate matters.

Personal Estate

If the deceased has no legal representative or next of kin in the country where they died, a U.S. consular officer may take responsibility for the personal estate of the deceased U.S. citizen, subject to local law. The consular officer may take possession of personal items, such as jewelry, documents, and clothing. The officer inventories these items and follows instructions from the legal representative or next of kin regarding their disposition.[2]

---

[2] Bureau of Consular Affairs, "Death Abroad," U.S. Department of State (DOS), March 4, 2024. Available online. URL: https://travel.state.gov/content/travel/en/international-travel/while-abroad/death-abroad1.html. Accessed August 1, 2024.

Part 8 | Additional Help and Information

Chapter 57 | **Glossary of Terms Related to Travel Health**

accompanying: A type of visa in which family members travel with the principal applicant, (in immigrant visa cases, within six months of issuance of an immigrant visa to the principal applicant).

acute: A short-term, intense-health effect.

agent: In immigrant visa processing, the applicant selects a person who receives all correspondence regarding the case and pays the immigrant visa application processing fee. The agent can be the applicant, the petitioner, or another person selected by the applicant and listed on Form DS-261, Online Choice of Address and Agent.

antibiotics: Medicines that damage or kill bacteria and are used to treat some bacterial diseases.

antibodies: Molecules (also called "immunoglobulins") produced by a B cell in response to an antigen. When an antibody attaches to an antigen, it destroys the antigen.

anxiety: Feelings of fear, dread, and uneasiness that may occur as a reaction to stress. A person with anxiety may sweat, feel restless and tense, and have a rapid heartbeat. Extreme anxiety that happens often over time may be a sign of an anxiety disorder.

applicant (visa): A foreign citizen who is applying for a nonimmigrant or immigrant U.S. visa. The visa applicant may also be referred as a "beneficiary" for petition based visas.

This glossary contains terms excerpted from documents produced by several sources deemed reliable.

aspirin: A drug that reduces pain, fever, inflammation, and blood clotting. Aspirin belongs to the family of drugs called "nonsteroidal anti-inflammatory agents." It is also being studied in cancer prevention.

assessment: In health care, a process used to learn about a patient's condition. This may include a complete medical history, medical tests, a physical exam, a test of learning skills, tests to find out if the patient is able to carry out the tasks of daily living, a mental-health evaluation, and a review of social support and community resources available to the patient.

assistive device: A tool that helps a person with a disability to do a certain task. Examples are a cane, wheelchair, scooter, walker, hearing aid, or special bed.

asthma: A chronic medical condition where the bronchial tubes (in the lungs) become easily irritated.

blood transfusion: The administration of blood or blood products into a blood vessel.

blood: A tissue with red blood cells, white blood cells, platelets, and other substances suspended in fluid called "plasma." Blood takes oxygen and nutrients to the tissues, and carries away wastes.

cancer: A disease in which some of the body's cells grow uncontrollably and spread to other parts of the body.

cardiopulmonary: Of or relating to the heart and lungs.

cell: The individual unit that makes up the tissues of the body. All living things are made up of one or more cells.

chemotherapy: Treatment with drugs that kill cancer cells.

clinical trial: A type of research study that tests how well new medical approaches work in people. These studies test new methods of screening, prevention, diagnosis, or treatment of a disease; also called a "clinical study."

computed tomography (CT): A computerized x-ray imaging procedure in which a narrow beam of x-rays is aimed at a patient and quickly rotated around the body, producing signals that are processed by the machine's computer to generate cross-sectional images—or "slices"—of the body.

counseling: The process by which a professional counselor helps a person cope with mental or emotional distress, and understand and solve personal problems.

cure: To heal or restore health; a treatment to restore health.

depression: A mental condition marked by ongoing feelings of sadness, despair, loss of energy, and difficulty dealing with normal daily life. Other symptoms of depression include feelings of worthlessness and hopelessness, loss of pleasure in activities, changes in eating or sleeping habits, and thoughts of death or suicide. Depression can affect anyone, and can be successfully treated. Depression affects 15 to 25 percent of cancer patients and up to one-third of the people who have a chronic illness.

diagnosis: The process of identifying a disease by the signs and symptoms.

drug: Any substance, other than food, that is used to prevent, diagnose, treat, or relieve symptoms of a disease or abnormal condition. Also refers to a substance that alters mood or body function, or that can be habit-forming or addictive, especially a narcotic.

epidemic: A disease outbreak that affects many people in a region at the same time.

homeless: People from countries that do not have a U.S. Embassy or Consulate where they can apply for immigrant visas are homeless. For example, the U.S. government does not have an embassy in Iran. Residents of Iran are "homeless" for visa purposes.

immunity: Protection from germs.

infection: Invasion and growth of germs in the body. The germs may be bacteria, viruses, yeast, fungi, or other microorganisms. Infections can begin anywhere in the body and may spread all through it. An infection can cause fever and other health problems, depending on where it occurs in the body.

inpatient: A person who is hospitalized for at least one night to receive treatment or participate in a study.

living will: A type of legal advance directive in which a person describes specific treatment guidelines that are to be followed by health-care providers if she or he becomes terminally ill and cannot communicate. A living will usually has instructions about whether to use aggressive medical treatment to keep a person alive such as cardiopulmonary resuscitation (CPR), artificial nutrition, or use of a respirator.

mental health: A person's overall psychological and emotional condition. Good mental health is a state of well-being in which a person is able to cope with everyday events, think clearly, be responsible, meet challenges, and have good relationships with others.

missionary work: Work performed for a religious organization to spread the faith (religion) and advance the principles and doctrines of the religion. Such work may include religious instruction, help for the elderly and needy, and proselytizing.

nutrition: The clinical practice concerned with nutrients and other substances contained in food and their action, interaction, and balance in relation to health and disease.

original document: The actual document that was issued when an authority recorded an event (e.g., birth, marriage, divorce, adoption, etc.).

orphan: A child who has no parents because of death, disappearance, desertion or abandonment of the parents. A child may also be considered an orphan if the child has an unwed mother, or a single living parent who cannot care for the child and has released her/him irrevocably (permanently) for adoption and emigration. Adoptive parents must make sure that a child meets the legal definition of an "orphan" before adopting a child from another country.

pandemic: An epidemic occurring over a very large geographic area.

post: U.S. Embassy, Consulate, or other diplomatic mission abroad. Not all U.S. Embassies, Consulates, and Missions are visa-issuing posts.

radiation: The emission of energy as electromagnetic waves or as moving subatomic particles, especially high-energy particles that cause ionization.

screening: Checking for disease when there are no symptoms.

side effect: A problem that occurs when treatment affects healthy tissues or organs. Some common side effects of cancer treatment are fatigue, pain, nausea, vomiting, decreased blood cell counts, hair loss, and mouth sores.

social service: A community resource that helps people in need. Services may include help getting to and from medical appointments, home delivery of medication and meals, in-home nursing care, help paying medical costs not covered by insurance, loaning medical equipment, and housekeeping help.

surgery: A medical specialty concerned with manual or operative procedures used in the diagnosis and treatment of diseases, injuries, or deformities. This specialty is usually responsible for the comprehensive management of the trauma victim and the critically ill surgical patient.

symptom: An indication that a person has a condition or disease. Some examples of symptoms are headache, fever, fatigue, nausea, vomiting, and pain.

ultrasound: An imaging test that uses sound waves to make pictures of organs, tissues, and other structures inside your body. It allows your health care provider to see into your body without surgery. Ultrasound is also called ultrasonography or sonography. Ultrasound images may be called sonograms.

Glossary of Terms Related to Travel Health

vaccine: A product made from very small amounts of weak or dead germs that can cause diseases—for example, viruses, bacteria, or toxins. It prepares your body to fight the disease faster and more effectively so you will not get sick. Vaccines are administered through needle injections, by mouth, and by aerosol.

visa: A citizen of a foreign country, wishing to enter the United States, generally must first obtain a visa, either a nonimmigrant visa for temporary stay, or an immigrant visa for permanent residence.

x-ray: A type of high-energy radiation. In low doses, x-rays are used to diagnose diseases by making pictures of the inside of the body.

Chapter 58 | **Directory of Organizations Providing Health and Safety Information for Travelers**

GOVERNMENT ORGANIZATIONS

Centers for Disease Control and Prevention (CDC)
1600 Clifton Rd., N.E.
Atlanta, GA 30329-4027
Toll-Free: 800-CDC-INFO
(800-232-4636)
Toll-Free TTY: 888-232-6348
Website: www.cdc.gov
Email: hrcs@cdc.gov

***Eunice Kennedy Shriver* National Institute of Child Health and Human Development (NICHD)**
P.O. Box 3006
Rockville, MD 20847
Toll-Free: 800-370-2943
Toll-Free Fax: 866-760-5947
Website: www.nichd.nih.gov

Email: NICHDInformation
ResourceCenter@
mail.nih.gov

Federal Trade Commission (FTC)
600 Pennsylvania Ave., N.W.
Washington, DC 20580
Phone: 202-326-2222
Website: www.ftc.gov

Office on Women's Health (OWH)
1101 Wootton Pkwy.
Rockville, MD 20852
Toll-Free: 800-994-9662
Phone: 202-690-7650
Fax: 202-205-2631
Website: www.womenshealth.gov
Email: womenshealth@hhs.gov

Resources in this chapter were compiled from several sources deemed reliable; all contact information was verified and updated in August 2024.

U.S. Bureau of Labor Statistics (BLS)

2 Massachusetts Ave., N.E.
Postal Sq., Bldg.
Washington, DC 20212-0001
Phone: 202-691-5200
Fax: 202-691-6444
Website: www.bls.gov

U.S. Department of Education (ED)

400 Maryland Ave., S.W.
Washington, DC 20202
Toll-Free: 800-USA-LEARN
(800-872-5327)
Phone: 202-401-2000
Website: www.ed.gov

U.S. Department of Health and Human Services (HHS)

200 Independence Ave., S.W.
Hubert H. Humphrey Bldg.
Washington, DC 20201
Toll-Free: 877-696-6775
Website: www.hhs.gov

U.S. Department of Transportation (DOT)

1200 New Jersey Ave., S.E.
Washington, DC 20590
Toll-Free: 855-368-4200
Phone: 202-366-4000
Website: www.transportation.gov

U.S. Environmental Protection Agency (EPA)

1200 Pennsylvania Ave., N.W.
Washington, DC 20460
Phone: 202-564-4700
Website: www.epa.gov

U.S. Food and Drug Administration (FDA)

10903 New Hampshire Ave.
Silver Spring, MD 20993-0002
Toll-Free: 888-INFO-FDA
(888-463-6332)
Phone: 301-796-8240
Website: www.fda.gov

PRIVATE ORGANIZATIONS

American Medical Association (AMA)

330 N. Wabash Ave., Ste. 39300
AMA Plz.
Chicago, IL 60611-5885
Phone: 312-464-4782
Website: www.ama-assn.org

The American Mosquito Control Association (AMCA)

One Capitol Mall, Ste. 800
Sacramento, CA 95814

Toll-Free: 888-626-0630
Website: www.mosquito.org
Email: amca@mosquito.org

Clean Water Fund

1444 Eye St., N.W., Ste. 400
Washington, DC 20005
Phone: 202-895-0420
Fax: 202-895-0438
Website: www.cleanwaterfund.org
Email: cwa@cleanwater.org

Food Allergy Research and Education (FARE)

7901 Jones Branch Dr., Ste. 240
McLean, VA 22102
Toll-Free: 800-929-4040
Phone: 703-691-3179
Fax: 703-691-2713
Website: www.fare.foodallergy.org

International Association for Medical Assistance to Travellers (IAMAT)

2430 Military Rd., Ste. 279
Niagara Falls, NY 14304
Phone: 716-754-4883
Website: www.iamat.org

International Cemetery, Cremation & Funeral Association (ICCFA)

107 Carpenter Dr., Ste. 100
Sterling, VA 20164
Toll-Free: 800-645-7700
Phone: 703-391-8400
Fax: 703-391-8416
Website: www.iccfa.com

International Food Protection Training Institute (IFPTI)

5220 Lovers Ln., Ste. LL-130
Portage, MI 49002
Phone: 269-488-3258
Website: www.ifpti.org

International Road Federation (IRF)

500 Montgomery St., Madison Pl.
5th Fl.
Alexandria, VA 22314
Phone: 703-535-1001
Fax: 703-535-1007
Website: www.irf.global
Email: info@IRF.global

Joint Commission International

One Renaissance Blvd., Ste. 401
Oakbrook Terrace, IL 60181
Phone: 630-268-7400
Website: www.
jointcommissioninternational.org
Email: JCRCustomerService@
jcrinc.com

National Center for Victims of Crime (NCVC)

P.O. Box 2770
Hyattsville, MD 20784
Phone: 202-467-8700
Website: www.victimsofcrime.org
Email: info@victimsofcrime.org

INDEX

INDEX

Page numbers followed by "n" refer to citation information; by "t" indicate tables; and by "f" indicate figures.

Index

Index

Index

Index

Index